A MARKETER'S GUIDE TO BRAND STRATEGY

ADVANCED TECHNIQUES FOR HEALTHCARE ORGANIZATIONS

CHRIS BEVOLO

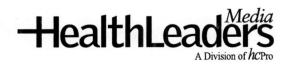

HealthLeaders *Media*
A Division of *hc*Pro

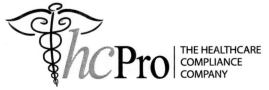

*hc*Pro | THE HEALTHCARE COMPLIANCE COMPANY

A Marketer's Guide to Brand Strategy: Advanced Techniques for Healthcare Organizations is published by HCPro, Inc.

Copyright © 2008 HCPro, Inc.

All rights reserved. Printed in the United States of America.   5   4   3   2   1

ISBN: 978-1-60146-163-6

HCPro, Inc., provides information resources for the healthcare industry.

HCPro, Inc., is not affiliated in any way with The Joint Commission, which owns the JCAHO and Joint Commission trademarks.

Chris Bevolo, Author

Gienna Shaw, Editor

Amy Anthony, Executive Editor

Matthew Cann, Group Publisher

Mike Mirabello, Senior Graphic Artist

Doug Ponte, Cover Designer

Audrey Doyle, Copyeditor

Alison Forman, Proofreader

Susan Darbyshire, Art Director

Darren Kelly, Books Production Supervisor

Claire Cloutier, Production Manager

Jean St. Pierre, Director of Operations

Advice given is general. Readers should consult professional counsel for specific legal, ethical, or clinical questions. Arrangements can be made for quantity discounts. For more information, contact:

HCPro, Inc.

P.O. Box 1168

Marblehead, MA 01945

Telephone: 800/650-6787 or 781/639-1872

Fax: 781/639-2982

E-mail: *customerservice@hcpro.com*

HCPro, Inc., is the parent company of Healthleaders Media.
Visit HCPro at its World Wide Web sites:
www.healthleadersmedia.com, www.hcpro.com, and *www.hcmarketplace.com*

Contents

Acknowledgments

Writing a book has been a lifelong dream of mine, and I'd like to thank the many people who made this dream possible.

First, thanks to Gienna Shaw, Amy Anthony, and HealthLeaders Media for providing the opportunity to publish my first book. Both Gienna and Amy were great to work with and provided terrific encouragement along the way. Thanks also to Heather West, our firm's public relations consultant and my right-hand woman in moving this book forward. Through spirited discussions over "ands" and "buts," Heather provided thorough and immediate response to all my questions and served as my first-line editor. The book would still be in the first-draft stage without her. Also, thanks to Chris Causey, my friend and branding sherpa, who always provided honest feedback and was not afraid to both trumpet the great points and call me on my BS.

Thanks to the instructors in my MBA program at the University of St. Thomas, who showed me that I could crank out text by the bucket load when required, and who helped give me a broader perspective on business and the world in general. My MBA cohort members—my journey with them ended just as I was beginning to work on this book—inspired me with their support and encouragement. I also want to acknowledge and thank the staff and associates at GeigerBevolo, who tolerated my absences while I was toiling away at the manuscript. Finally, thanks to all the clients whose branding endeavors afforded me frontline experience, along with all of the authors, experts, consultants, and others who have shaped my perspectives over the years. Thanks especially to those who shared with me their time and the information for the case studies in this book.

Finally, and most important of all, I want to thank my kids: Jackson, Julia, and Callie. They inspire me every day to always do more and to do better. This book is for them (though I'm sure they will find it way too boring). I love you each with all of my heart.

About the author

Chris Bevolo

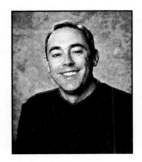 **Chris Bevolo** serves as owner and director of client strategy for GeigerBevolo, Inc., a healthcare branding firm based in Twin Cities, MN. He has 17 years of experience, focusing on leading the development of brand strategies and campaigns, patient experience strategies, and marketing campaigns for healthcare clients including Children's Hospitals & Clinics of Minnesota, Woodwinds Health Campus (Woodbury, MN), North Memorial Health Care (Robbinsdale, MN), Foote Health System (Jackson, MI), Hudson (WI) Hospital, Blue Cross and Blue Shield of Minnesota, and the Minnesota Hospital Association. He has been a keynote presenter and for a variety of organizations, has served as a judge in local and regional design and marketing competitions, and has published a number of articles and white papers. He is a member of the Minnesota Hospital Association, Minnesota Health Strategies and Communications Network, Society for Healthcare Strategy & Market Development, and International Association of Business Communicators. Chris received an MBA from the University of St. Thomas in Minneapolis, and his bachelor's degree in journalism and mass communications at Iowa State University.

Introduction

Brand: It's not a four-letter word

A few years ago, our branding firm, GeigerBevolo, Inc., was working with a large metropolitan health system on a strategic marketing campaign for its oncology service line. As part of the process, the marketing manager and I had scheduled a meeting with the organization's top exec to get his views on the campaign. He was enthusiastic and inspired—floating ideas for the marketing effort and pulling reports and articles from his files to share with us. But when I raised the issue of branding as it related to the independent physicians who were part of the service line, his mood changed. There was a moment of silence, and I'll never forget the look that crossed his face or the statement he issued next. "Branding," he said with disgust. "You can do whatever you want with that [expletive deleted]."

Although this kind of outright hatred for the concept of branding is probably rare, when it comes to embracing the strategy healthcare marketers constantly face challenges from their leaders and the rest of their organization. In the worst circumstances, healthcare leaders view branding as worthless—a fluffy marketing term that has no value in the world of healthcare. More often, branding is misunderstood, mistakenly identified as an organization's advertising or its logo.

More than just a pretty logo

Branding, of course, is much more than the visual identity, name, or advertising campaign of a hospital or health system. Branding is a strategy that reaches every corner of an organization to transform behaviors, decisions, and entire cultures. It's a strategy that has been employed in other industries for years, but has only recently begun to find its place in the healthcare provider market. Significant market forces, such as increased competition and the growing empowerment of consumers, make branding even more critical to the long-term success of healthcare providers.

Healthcare organizations have been changing their visual identities and running brand campaigns for years. But the true essence of branding is living the brand. Logos and ads are means to translate brands and, if created effectively, to reinforce them through style and clarity. However, brands fundamentally are built through the products, services, and experiences that organizations provide throughout the years to their markets. Of course, this is the hard work of branding—moving an organization to fulfill its brand promise.

Embrace your brand

You may not think about your brand very often (or, as in the earlier example of our executive, you might think of branding in a negative way). Regardless, all organizations do have a brand. So, the question isn't whether you want to have a brand, but whether you want to deliberately manage and build it. I wrote this book for those leaders who are ready to embrace branding as a strategy, but are unsure where to start, what specific steps to take, or how to make their brand strategy stick.

Readers will find strategies and tips for truly building brands, and examples of how other healthcare providers have embraced branding. To help provide a foundation for that work, I've also included a solid background on the concept of branding. I'll answer the following questions:

- What is branding?
- Why is branding valuable?
- How is branding related to marketing, strategy, and vision?
- How is branding different for healthcare providers?

How to use this book

I've written this book in a linear fashion, outlining the basics of branding before exploring the harder work of building brands. If your organization is just starting down the branding path, you can (and should!) read this book from cover to cover to get a complete overview and context of the concept of brand strategy. If your organization has already begun to travel along the branding path, you'll find that this book is divided into four sections that allow you to jump to the topic that's most relevant to you.

Looking for direction

If you're convinced of the value of branding but others in the organization, including leaders, physicians, and other stakeholders, are not on board, I suggest you start with the first part of this book, which discusses why branding as a strategy is so important to healthcare organizations.

Starting down the path

If you're convinced of the value of branding and are working to get your stakeholders on board but you need more information about where to start, or if you are concerned about how it will work in your organization, you might want to start with the second section of the book, which discusses the ins and outs of branding and brand strategy.

Hitting your stride

If you're up to speed on branding, have everyone on board, and are ready to proactively begin to manage or build your organization's brand, start with the third section of the book, on building brands.

Coming out of the woods

If you're already blazing trails in your organization but want to go even further or are looking for specific ideas to make your effort more successful, turn to the fourth section of this book, the case studies. Here you'll find advice and inspiration from healthcare organizations that are doing some of the best work on brand strategy in the business.

Regardless of your branding experience, your philosophy about its value, and the stage of your organization's brand journey, all four sections of the book will prove useful to readers who want to fully understand the power of building a successful brand.

A few caveats

There are a few things to keep in mind when reading this book. First, I wrote this book from a definite point of view. I fully believe in the power of branding to reshape organizations and position them effectively for long-term success. This book will make that case. Readers won't find an intellectually objective debate on the pros and cons of branding—this book is most definitely pro. With that said, however, I'm a big believer in the premise behind the book *The Wisdom of Crowds,* by James Surowiecki. Although I'm bringing my beliefs and biases to the table, those beliefs have been shaped by numerous others— speakers, authors, experts, competitors, and clients. This book liberally leverages the expertise of these sources and others who are better informed and more experienced in building brands than I. A thousand heads, in this case, are better than one.

Second, branding as a strategy in its truest form is relatively new to the world of healthcare. Generously speaking, branding as a strategy entered the lexicon of leadership in only the past decade. Even now, most health systems, hospitals, and clinics have no true branding strategy. Thus, stories of healthcare provider organizations that successfully have implemented a branding strategy are rare. Add to that the complex nature of measuring successful branding efforts and you'll understand why it takes years for brand strategies to take hold and show benefit. Nevertheless, understanding the value of branding and learning from those who have started down the path should prove invaluable to other organizations that believe in branding.

Finally, there's no doubt that branding is extraordinarily difficult to pull off. It took McDonald's at least 10 years to build a national brand, and it took Starbucks more than 20 years. Similarly, it took such healthcare giants as the Mayo Clinic, Johns Hopkins Medicine, and the Cleveland Clinic decades to build their brands. This stuff doesn't happen overnight.

Of course, your goal may not be to create a brand that is recognized and valued nationally, and the time frame in which you expect results is likely less than 20 years. Nevertheless, you shouldn't pursue branding lightly, as the roadblocks and pitfalls are numerous. It takes strategic focus, discipline, patience, and a lot of luck. But a successful brand strategy can reap countless benefits, bringing years of success and security. Look again at the short list of healthcare organizations in the preceding paragraph—who wouldn't want to be next on that list?

Why build brands?

Before launching into an explanation of how to build brands, or even a description of what defines a brand, it's often helpful to address why branding is an important strategy for healthcare organizations. It may seem a bit backward to outline the value of branding before defining the term. However, I've found that before "nonbelievers" will commit to learning about branding, they need a taste of its power and the results it can bring to an organization.

The benefits of branding

The benefits of branding are well documented but often have to be revisited when a branding initiative is under consideration in a healthcare organization. In his book, *Building Strong Brands*, author and brand guru David Aaker cites 17 different ways that a brand creates value for organizations, including reduced marketing costs, easier extension of products and services, customer loyalty, ability to charge higher prices, attraction of new customers, and more. These reasons and benefits of branding are known among healthcare marketing professionals, but they're not often understood or accepted by leaders and others within the organization. Marketing professionals who cite the benefits of branding often hear the following questions:

- What proof do we have that branding has these effects?
- What does branding mean for our bottom line?

The resulting discussion of the value of branding frequently takes place on two levels: branding's impact on the individual consumer and branding's impact on the organization as a whole.

This is your brain on brands

At its most elemental level, branding seeks to change our minds—literally. In his book on understanding the mind of the market, *How Customers Think,* author Gerald Zaltman outlines how the unconscious mind is shaped from millions of inputs from our environment.

"Ninety-five percent of thinking takes place in our unconscious minds," he writes, "that wonderful, if messy, stew of memories, emotions, thoughts, and other cognitive processes we're not aware of or that we can't articulate."

The ongoing saga of Pepsi versus Coke has given us ample evidence that supports the impact of branding on the unconscious minds of consumers. In a 2000 article for the magazine *Advertising Age,* columnist Bob Garfield took

Pepsi to task for reinstituting Pepsi's famous taste test, the Pepsi Challenge, as a marketing strategy. He based his argument on the very essence of the value of brand, which often overrides fact or reality in the minds of consumers. "Taste preference is all well and good, but it has very little to do with brand preference," Garfield writes. "Pepsi should understand that, too, because although more people preferred the taste of Pepsi over Coca-Cola in 1975, and 1980, and 1985, and in 1990, and in 1995 and, no doubt, 2000, more people continue to buy Coke." Pepsi, Garfield says, has repeatedly failed the true Pepsi Challenge, which is to alter consumer perceptions, to broaden the Pepsi audience, to generate the same level of emotion as its main competitor, and to be not merely liked, but loved by the consumer.

More recently, technology has provided further evidence of the impact of branding using soda preference as the testing ground. Now, new scanning technologies such as functional magnetic resonance imaging (fMRI) machines can measure the impact of branding on actual brain function. Researchers at the Baylor College of Medicine used this technology during a blind taste test of Pepsi and Coke. After receiving a taste of a soda while in the fMRI machine, participants showed strong activity in the reward areas of the brain, which are associated with pleasure and satisfaction. When the researchers conducted a blind taste test, participants were evenly split in their preference between Coke and Pepsi. However, when participants were told when they were sampling Coke or Pepsi, 75% stated a preference for Coke. In addition to the reward area of their brains, activity was found in the medial prefrontal cortex and hippocampus, which are areas responsible for memory. As the lead researcher noted, this demonstrated that the brand alone has perceived value in the brain system above and beyond the desire for the taste of the soda itself—thus scientific proof of the power of brand.

Finally, another great way to understand the power of brand at the individual level lies in the fact that consumers will consistently pay more money for a trusted brand. How can Tylenol remain profitable by selling the same pain reliever at twice the cost of a generic brand? People will pay twice as much because they believe Tylenol is better, despite the fact that it's the same formula as a generic. Such is the power of the Tylenol brand.

Branding and the bottom line

Understanding the impact of branding at the neural level is important, but it rarely suffices as an answer to the hospital CFO who demands proof that branding will add value before he or she puts funds into it. I'll address measurement of individual brands later in the book, but there's plenty of proof that branding impacts an organization's financial success.

Every year, national business publications such as *BusinessWeek* release their lists of the top national and international brands. The August 6, 2007 *BusinessWeek* article "Best Global Brands" ranks Coca-Cola first, with a monetary brand value of $65,324,000. The magazine uses a complicated formula to determine this brand value, isolating corporate earnings that can be tied directly to brand and stripping away all other factors. In essence, brand value equates to goodwill, the line item on a balance sheet that often corresponds to the highest-valued asset. This asset is monetized when a company merges or is sold. For example, when Philip Morris bought Kraft Foods, the purchase price of $12.9 billion was more than four times the amount of Kraft's tangible assets, demonstrating the significant value attributed to the Kraft brand.

Along with a base value to organizations, research shows that stronger brands bring greater value. For example, a study on branding by The Conference Board notes that total revenues for companies with highly successful branding strategies were 11% higher than other companies over a five-year period, and those companies' stock valuations were 54% higher than other companies'. And according to "What Price Reputation?" in the July 9, 2007 issue of *BusinessWeek*, a company's brand reputation can account for much of the 30%–70% gap between its book value and its market capitalization. The article spotlights researchers who are developing new methods for measuring the impact of branding on stock prices. For example, based on the research, brand strength is demonstrated to have a significant impact on the differences in stock price between rival companies, such as Procter & Gamble versus Unilever, or Exxon Mobil versus Royal Dutch Shell.

But does it apply to healthcare?

The evidence presented in the preceding section revolves around nonhealthcare industries, products, and services. Can that evidence be extrapolated to healthcare providers for those who need further proof of the value of branding?

Many believe the healthcare industry is unique, starting with its mission of providing medical care to the sick and injured. In fact, given this mission, many in the United States prefer to categorize providers as charities rather than businesses.

Whether for-profit or not-for-profit, the vast majority of healthcare providers are part of a market-driven industry, forced to compete for resources and customers with others in the same business. Barring a radical shift to a government-run system, healthcare providers must compete, win business, and take in more money than they spend. Given those realities, they must seek the most effective strategies available to achieve those goals. The fact that there is little research proving the value of branding in healthcare provider organizations does not mean it doesn't provide value. Rather, the reason for this lack of data is that the strategy is so new in this industry.

Many healthcare leaders believe in the strategies espoused by Jim Collins in his best-selling book, *Good to Great*. In a follow-up monograph titled "Good to Great and the Social Sectors," Collins uses brand building as a key element in the flywheel concept. He explains that if organizations follow all of the key strategies of great companies, the effect is like a flywheel, where success breeds more success in an ongoing, positive cycle.

"Whereas in business, the key driver in the flywheel is the link between financial success and capital resources, I'd like to suggest that a key link in the social sectors is brand reputation—built upon tangible results and emotional share of heart—so that potential supporters believe not only in your mission, but in your capacity to deliver on that mission," he writes.

Although healthcare providers face many challenges in building brands that are unique to the industry, the value of brand-building is clear. In the end, branding wields power wherever there is choice in a market. And as we'll see in Chapter 2, choice is just one driver that makes branding a critical strategy for today's healthcare leaders.

References

David Aakers. *Building Strong Brands* (Simon & Schuster: 2002), p. 9.

Gerald Zaltman. *How Customers Think* (Harvard Business School Press: 2003), p. 9.

Bob Garfield. "Pepsi may win Challenge, but loses most crucial test." *Advertising Age*, March 27, 2000.

Alice Park. "Marketing to your mind." *Time Magazine*, January 29, 2007.

David Kiley. "The 100 Top Brands." *BusinessWeek*, August 6, 2007, p. 59.

Paul Stobard (Ed.). *Brand Power* (NYU Press: 1994).

Kathryn Troy. "Managing the Corporate Brand." The Conference Board (1998), p. 7.

The time is right for healthcare branding

As mentioned earlier, branding as a strategy is relatively new to the healthcare provider industry, having only really come into play over the past decade or so. To understand how the industry is shifting, it helps to consider another industry that went through a similar shift: the banking industry.

Consumerism and the death of bankers' hours

In today's world of ATMs, online banking, and Sunday hours at the local bank branch, many people have forgotten all about the term *bankers' hours* or its origin—the fact that many banks closed at 3 p.m. weekdays and were closed weekends. For the course of most of this nation's history, banks were pretty much the only choice for financial services, facing little competition for a consumer's savings. Banks knew there were few other ways for consumers to deposit, save, or invest money, and they acted accordingly.

Originally, there may have been valid reasons for banks to keep shorter hours. But by the 1970s and 1980s, it was still a common practice to close early, despite an obvious change in consumer demand. Why were these inconvenient bankers' hours maintained? Maybe because banks knew consumers had little choice to go elsewhere. However, when deregulation arrived in the early 1980s, and the stock market boom of the 1990s followed, banks became only one of many options consumers had for saving and investing. As a result, banks had to learn how to compete and market their services, and how to provide convenience and deliver better service to their customers.

Healthcare providers today are in much the same boat as bankers were in the early 1980s. As with the banking industry before them, healthcare providers are now being forced to consider branding as a strategic weapon. But why now? The shift in the healthcare provider industry didn't come from government deregulation. Instead, branding has begun to emerge thanks to the intersection of two major market forces that have the potential to drive dramatic change in the industry: the rise of competition and the consumer.

Force one: The rise of competition

Until the 1970s, "competition" was not on the strategic radar for most healthcare providers. With a few exceptions, healthcare providers adhered to ideology attributed to Sir William Osler: "The practice of medicine is an art, not a trade; a calling, not a business." This mindset began to change after the HMO Act of 1973, though real market pressures didn't begin to hit until the 1980s with the advent of managed care. Suddenly, patient flow was restricted, and healthcare providers had to consider ways to keep patient volumes up. Most hospitals and health systems didn't even have marketing departments until the 1980s. During the 1980s and 1990s, many healthcare organizations grew in size and scope, many large national chains were created (such as Humana and HCA), and physician-owned hospitals and specialty clinics became more prominent. All of this ushered in a new, highly competitive atmosphere.

In more recent years, new types of competition have entered the fray. Consider the rise of mini clinics, which you can now find in Wal-Mart, Target, Walgreens, and many other major retailers. Or RevolutionHealth, the healthcare company launched by entrepreneur Steve Case, former CEO and founder of America Online. Case started RevolutionHealth with more than $500 million of his own money and a mission to "revolutionize" the delivery of healthcare. Consider, too, the overseas options increasingly available to U.S. patients, where care is delivered in a beautiful locale for a fraction of the cost and with obstensibly the same level of quality. As Thomas Friedman warns in his best-selling book, *The World Is Flat*, upon his realization of the potential impact of globalization on America, "The global competitive playing field was being leveled . . . As I came to this realization, I was filled with both excitement and dread."

These entrants represent a new breed of competitor for the traditional healthcare organization: those who seek to build businesses in healthcare from outside the industry. Successful companies and entrepreneurs from outside the medical world are turning their eyes to healthcare in a major way. The healthcare industry as a whole is the largest in the United States in terms of gross domestic product, with more than $2 trillion in spending in 2005, according to the U.S. Department of Health and Human Services. Given that, and the vast inefficiencies and poor service levels many attribute to traditional healthcare providers, it's no wonder that business leaders from other industries see opportunity in healthcare. Not only do they want to deliver healthcare services, but they believe they can do so in superior ways and for less money. Because these new entrants often bring sophisticated marketing expertise, a spirit of innovation, an inherent "consumer perspective," and deep pockets to the market, traditional providers will be under more pressure to adopt more sophisticated strategies themselves.

Whether it's an overseas surgery center, a new physician-owned speciality clinic, an alternative-medicine store at the mall, or the hospital across town, healthcare providers are facing increasing competition. More competition makes it harder to find, attract, and keep customers, which is one reason branding is now a hot strategy for provider organizations.

Force two: The rise of the consumer

Consumerism has been a watchword for healthcare providers for a number of years, but the ultimate impact of this movement has yet to be truly felt. Many factors are leading to more empowered healthcare consumers. The first is an increase in choices for care. As noted previously, the more competition in the market, the more choice for consumers. With more choices, consumers will be exposed to better options, raising their expectations and thereby raising the bar for traditional providers of care.

In addition, healthcare consumers are much better educated now than they were even a decade ago, thanks to the Internet and other media outlets. With access to more information, consumers are empowered to understand and direct their own medical care. Consumers can now simply sit down at their home computers and search for information on any ailment, physician, or healthcare system. The number of Web sites dedicated to providing information on healthcare providers, related to quality, price, and service, is growing every year. Consumers can turn to payers such as Blue Cross and Blue Shield, companies such as HealthGrades, organizations such as LeapFrog, national and state government entities such as the Centers for Medicare & Medicaid Services, hospital associations, or the providers themselves for information on how to value a particular healthcare choice.

But perhaps most important is the fact that the proliferation of consumer-driven healthcare will force individuals to shoulder more of the financial burden of their own healthcare. In essence, the average consumer has more skin in the game, and the impact of that shift could be dramatic. Of course, consumer spending on healthcare has already affected the industry. Thanks in large part to the economic boom that started in the mid-1990s, consumers have spent more discretionary income on elective health-related services, such as cosmetic surgery, alternative medicine, and more. Many hospitals and health systems have responded with retail strategies, cosmetic surgery centers, and other initiatives to capitalize on this shift. But now consumers are also increasingly spending their own money on nonelective health services, which make up the bulk of a provider's revenue stream.

Consumer-driven health plans are usually defined as Health Reimbursement Accounts, Health Savings Accounts, high-deductible insurance plans, or other policies that offer lower premiums in return for enrollees paying more out-ofpocket funds up-front for their care. The idea is that with more of their own money on the line, consumers will make smarter decisions about their care, which should lead to more efficient use of medical services and overall lower expenditures in healthcare. Participation in consumer-driven health plans has risen from about 7,000 in 2001 to an estimated six million in early 2006 to more than 10 million in January 2007.

As consumers spend more of their own money for care, they will begin to apply value factors in their decision-making as they do for other significant purchases. For example, most consumers—either explicitly or unconsciously— consider value factors such as price, quality, service, experience, and reputation when considering a new-car purchase or picking up a new computer for the home. In the past, with little or no money on the line, patients were much less likely to consider these values in choosing their care. It is much easier to forgive poor service, a bad location, or a grumpy doctor when your investment is a $10 copayment. But now, with $1,000, $3,000, or even $10,000 of their own money on the line, many patients will want to ensure that they are "getting their money's worth," which makes building a strong brand essential.

How much of an impact could consumer-driven healthcare have on consumer decision-making? The answer may not be known for some time, but here's one analogy that puts the situation into perspective. In 2005, Hurricane Katrina devastated New Orleans and the Gulf Coast, and before cleanup could even begin, the region was threatened by Hurricane Rita. Anderson Cooper, the suave and ubiquitous correspondent from CNN, was reporting from Corpus Christi, TX, which was directly in the path of the new storm. As he stood on the shoreline of the Gulf of Mexico at dusk, he pointed out to the darkening skies, then down to the water's edge, where the waves were lapping up to his feet. Fully dramatizing the occasion, he showed how the waves were getting higher and higher, a certain portend of the coming monster storm.

He could have just been reporting on a windy day, as the waves were really nothing out of the ordinary at that time. But that scene is where the industry stands today relative to consumer-driven healthcare. We can see a storm on the horizon, and hospitals, health systems, and others in the industry are just beginning to feel its effects. If this market trend is indeed a "Category 5" storm and it makes a direct hit, it has the potential to turn the industry upside down.

For example, can you imagine online auctions for surgery? Full pricing menus at hospitals? Clinics with different entrances, one for standard patients and one for "club members"? Who knows whether any of these concepts will come to fruition, but the point is that consumer-driven trends could have a profound effect on healthcare in the United States. Of course, the storm could downgrade into a Category One, or it could miss north or south. Maybe the changes will have less of an impact than some predict. But either way, even the threat of the change is altering how healthcare providers must think about their businesses.

Thirty years ago, a patient was told by her doctor to go to the local hospital, and that's what she did. There were few alternatives, and the patient was un-likely to know about them and had little incentive to consider another choice. Now patients have many more choices, both physical and virtual, and have more information on those choices than they know what to do with. Their expectations are greater, their demands are higher, and their financial incentives are clearer. All of this leads to a significant challenge for healthcare providers: How do you convince that patient you are the best choice on the market? Because there are more competitors and because consumers are demanding more, healthcare providers must be smart about providing value that markets desire, and differentiating that value from others in the market. That makes branding more relevant today than ever before for traditional providers of healthcare, as differentiation is a cornerstone of effective brand-building. In his book on branding, *Zag*, author Marty Neumeier starts by building a case for differentiation, with the first paragraph setting the stage: "An overabundance of look-alike products and me-too services is forcing customers to search for something, anything, to help them separate the winners from the clutter."

In surveying the landscape of hospital and health-system marketing, the prevalence of "look-alike" and "me-too" strategies, tactics, and communications is epidemic. In healthcare, traditional differentiation takes the form of patient satisfaction results, a new piece of imaging technology, a specialist's certification, or another smiling patient testimonial. Using branding as a long-term strategy will force your organization to move beyond these basic tactics and to plan how it will stand out from the competition and compel consumers to turn to your service offerings.

Reference

Cromwick, Hughes, Paul Root, and Sarah Roehrig. Business Economics, April 1, 2007.

3

The ins and outs of branding

Now that we've outlined why brands have value in today's market for health-care provider organizations, it's time to back up a step and answer the question: What exactly is a brand?

In 1964, Supreme Court Justice Potter Stewart explained the courts' ruling on obscenity with the classic line, "I know it when I see it." For many, branding holds the same sort of undefinable quality. Ask 10 people to define branding as it relates to the nonhealthcare sector and you'll get 10 different answers. In healthcare, you'll probably get 20.

Over the years, a number of branding experts have attempted to define the term *brand*. The word itself comes from the practice of applying a red-hot iron "brand" to a steer to mark the animal's ownership. Thus, in a classic interpretation, your brand is your name. For example, Procter & Gamble produces five brands of laundry detergent, including Tide and Cheer. But consider again the cattle ranch scenario. Let's say two ranchers, Rancher Tom and Rancher Bob, owned cattle in the town of Westville. To ensure that they could tell their steers apart, each used a unique brand to identify their cattle. Tom used a *T* and Bob used a *B*. Thus, all the cattle in the market were branded either *T* for Tom's cattle or *B* for Bob's cattle.

But then consider that Tom was a better rancher and understood how to raise cattle better than Bob. He gave them better shelter, fed them higher-quality feed, and kept them healthier. So, when Tom brought his cattle to market, they were usually bigger than Bob's and provided more meat. Over time, the buyers at the market noted these differences and began to pay more for Tom's cattle. Now the letter *T* served more than identification purposes. It was a symbol to the market—a symbol of better value and of better cattle. Tom had established a better brand than Bob, and he was able to charge more money for that brand, even when one of his cows was the same size as one of Bob's. The mere fact that one cow had a *T* brand gave it more value in the eyes of the market than the cow with a *B*. Today, most experts agree that brand is defined as the value behind a product, service, or company name—as defined by the consumer.

Scott Bedbury spent seven years as head of advertising at Nike. He helped to launch the famous "Just Do It" campaign and to build the well-regarded Nike brand. Following that, Bedbury was senior vice president of marketing at Starbucks, where building a powerful brand was a core philosophy. In his book, *A New Brand World*, Bedbury describes the term *brand* in this way:

A brand is the sum of the good, the bad, the ugly, and the off-strategy. It is defined by your best product as well as your worst product. It is defined by award-winning advertising as well as by the God-awful ads that somehow slipped through the cracks, got approved, and, not surprisingly, sank into oblivion. It is defined by the accomplishments of your best employee—the shining star in the company who can do no wrong—as well as by the mishaps of the worst hire that you ever made. It is also defined by your receptionist and the music your customers are subjected to when placed on hold. For every grand and finely worded public statement by the CEO, the brand is also defined by derisory consumer comments overheard in the hallway or in a chat room on the Internet. Brands are sponges for content, for images, for fleeting feelings. They become psychological concepts held in the minds of the public, where they may stay forever. As such you can't entirely control a brand. At best you only guide and influence it.

A more concise definition comes from Marty Neumeier, in his book, *The Brand Gap*:

A brand is a person's gut feeling about a product, service or company. It's a gut feeling because we're all emotional, intuitive beings, despite our best efforts to be rational. It's a person's gut feeling, because in the end the brand is defined by individuals, not by companies, markets or the so-called general public. Each person creates his or her own version of it. While companies can't control this process, they can influence it by communicating the qualities that make this product different than that product. When enough individuals arrive at the same gut feeling, a company can be said to have a brand. In other words, a brand is not what you say it is. It's what they say it is.

As you can tell from these two definitions by highly respected brand experts, the idea of brand can be fairly fuzzy. One consistent theme is that brand resides in the mind of the consumer. That is, the consumer defines your brand, not you. Many experts even break brand down to the simplest of emotional differentiation: Do consumers feel positive or negative about your organization as a whole? In his book, *Building Strong Brands*, author David Aakers likens a brand to a "mental box":

> A brand such as Mr. Goodwrench is much like a "box" in someone's head. As information about GM service programs is received, a person will file it away in the box labeled Mr. Goodwrench. After time passes, little in the box might be retrievable. The person knows, however, if it is heavy or light. He or she also knows in which room it is stored—the room with the positive boxes (that is, objects that have earned positive feelings and attitudes) or the one with the negative boxes.

Have you ever had the experience of being at a cocktail party or your kid's soccer game, and someone mentions a name that you can't quite place? You know you've heard of this person, but you can't remember exactly who he is. However, your internal radar is flashing and your senses tell you that something isn't quite right about this person, even if you can't put a finger on it. A few hours later, it hits you out of the blue: "Oh, Tom Smith! I remember him—he was fired for embezzlement from the bank my cousin works at." That, at its most base level, is your brand value of Tom Smith, which provided you with a gut-level reaction to Tom before you could remember exactly who he was.

So, where does this leave us in defining *brand*? A brand is the value, the emotion, and the reputation a consumer gives any organization, product, or service. All companies, products, and services have a brand, whether they know it or not, and regardless of whether they deliberately set out to build one. It's not a question of whether you want a brand. You have one whether you like it or not. The question is how proactive you will be in shaping it.

Branding is how an organization goes about trying to influence how audiences value its organization, product, or service. Branding seeks to manage all possible touch points with a consumer to have that consumer think and feel about a company, product, or service in a given way. It can influence all aspects of a business and shape decisions in every part of the marketing continuum, from product development to service delivery to communications. It's with this definition of branding that many nonmarketers become confused. They see branding as communications-oriented, when in fact communications is just one component of branding. Branding is first and foremost about living a brand. Consider some of the ways a hospital potentially builds its brand with a patient who comes in for a routine checkup. The patient (and his or her family) will notice some or all of the following:

- The convenience of parking at the hospital and whether there is a cost
- The cleanliness of the bathrooms
- The level of eye contact from the staff member at the information desk
- The simplicity of the way-finding
- The length of the wait before an appointment
- The friendliness of the nurse during a blood pressure check

- The amount of time a doctor spends in the exam room
- The clarity of the bill that arrives 15 days later

This, of course, represents only a tiny fraction of the touch points one patient may encounter, but note that none of these are related to communications tactics. This shouldn't be surprising. Consider the brands you value. How many of them have been based solely, or even primarily, on the ads you see on television or the brochures you read? In fact, a brand is typically shaped by all of the following:

- Product or service experience
- Customer service
- Price
- Environment
- Reputation
- Word-of-mouth
- Marketing, communications, public relations
- Corporate identity

The components of brand strategy

To consider branding as a strategy, it helps to define some of its key components. Brand strategy is a generic term for a high-level, overarching strategy for leveraging branding as a discipline for meeting long-term organizational goals. A brand strategy is a guiding blueprint for how an organization wants to brand itself for the future. At their most basic, brand strategies often contain three key elements (note that differing labels may be used, with slight variations on content, depending on the approach or source):

- Brand promise: the overriding descriptor of the brand an organization wants its audiences to hold in their minds and hearts about the organization

- Brand attributes: the values or "essence" of the desired brand

- Brand embodiment: ways in which an organization demonstrates and communicates its brand

In addition to outlining these concepts, a brand strategy may also provide the rationale for the organization's decisions regarding brand-naming, hierarchy, visual identity, and more.

Brand embodiment

Of all the elements of branding, brand embodiment is the most vital. It defines all the ways in which your organization provides value to your customers, how it lives the brand. Brand embodiment is synonymous with phrases such as "brand experience," "living the brand," and "delivering on a brand promise." Brand embodiment is critical because no matter how unique your name, how sophisticated your strategy, or how creative your communications, if you can't deliver a great brand experience, nothing else will matter. In fact, one of the biggest mistakes healthcare organizations make is to move too fast or too far in promoting their services without having a brand experience that lives up to the hype.

I once worked with the CEO of a health system who lamented the poor reputation of a key service line. That reputation was earned through years of bad service and poor clinical outcomes. The CEO called upon the director of marketing to solve this problem. "We need an ad campaign to start fixing our bad reputation," he said. That, of course, is backward. You can repair a poor reputation only by fixing what's broken: service and clinical quality. Compelling new patients to try out a bad experience will actually do more harm than good.

In his book, *Zag*, Neumeier stresses the critical role that experience plays in brand-building:

> *Every brand is built with experiences, whether the brand is a company, product or service and whether it serves individuals or businesses. The key is to craft those experiences so they create delight for the people who determine the meaning and value of your brand—your customers.*

The best proof that brand comes before communication comes from Starbucks, a company that built itself into one of the best-known and most-valued brands in the world without, initially at least, any advertising at all. The same holds true for the Mayo Clinic, perhaps the world's most recognized and respected healthcare brand, which began to run its first consumer advertising only recently.

Fully embodying a compelling and consistent brand is usually the most difficult part of branding, the Holy Grail of branding. Later in the book, I'll explore how healthcare organizations can tackle this significant challenge.

Brand identity

Brand identity is a broad term for the identifying elements of a brand, including brand name and corporate identity. The definition of the term *brand name* would seem to speak for itself, but depending on an organization's brand hierarchy (discussed shortly) different brand names within an organization may hold different brand value in the market. For example, what's the difference in your mind between a Toyota Corolla, a Toyota Prius, and a Toyota Camry? Organizations often invest thousands of dollars in renaming to help bolster a brand, but a wise sage once told me that the name doesn't make the brand, the brand makes the name.

For example, think of the brand cachet of McDonald's. On its own, does the name do anything to further an understanding or valuing of the product offering? Would that organization start from scratch to build the world's largest hamburger chain and choose McDonald's as the best name for the brand? This bit of wisdom holds true with so many other brands as well, such as Google, Xerox, and of course, the Mayo Clinic. A name shouldn't confuse consumers or serve as an obstacle for use, but always remember that what goes into a name is what matters.

Corporate identity

Corporate identity is often used to describe all elements of an organization's visual symbolism, including logomark (a symbol or icon), namemark (how a name is treated visually), signatures (how distinct names and/or logomarks are combined visually), colors, typefaces, and more. Although this term usually applies to visual elements, many organizations also consider other senses when building branded identities. For example, Harley-Davidson trademarked the roar of its engine, and Metro-Goldwyn-Mayer the roar of a lion. NBC trademarked its distinctive three-note chime, and Intel claims its own signature "ding" as a registered trademark. The shape of Coca-Cola's bottle is registered, as is the uniquely pink color of Owens Corning's insulation. Smells are the newest battle on the brand frontier. In Europe, the smell of freshly cut grass has been trademarked by a company that makes tennis balls.

Brand hierarchy

Brand hierarchy defines how brand names are structured throughout an organization, and hierarchy can have a significant impact on branding for an organization. Traditionally, there are three types of brand name hierarchies: unified branding, endorsed branding, and product branding.

Unified branding is when an organization uses one brand name to market all elements of that organization. Examples include Wells Fargo, IBM, and Volvo. In healthcare, examples include the Mayo Clinic and Provena Health in Chicago. The unified branding strategy is also known as corporate branding, umbrella branding, and master branding.

Endorsed branding is when an organization has a group of companies, products, or services with individual brand names that are supported with the overall organization name. Examples include General Motors and Kellogg's. Chevrolet is a General Motors brand and Frosted Flakes and Fruit Loops are individual brands endorsed by the Kellogg's master brand. In healthcare, Allina Hospitals & Clinics in Minnesota is an example of an endorsed branding strategy (Abbott Northwestern Hospital and United Hospital are both part of the Allina Hospital & Clinics system). As noted, the Mayo Clinic follows a unified branding philosophy. However, the organization's broader system of acquired hospitals and clinics, the Mayo Health System, follows an endorsed hierarchy. For example, the Albert Lea Medical Center is part of the Mayo Health System. (Conceivably, this was done to protect the valuable Mayo Clinic brand from possible dilution from the acquisition of lesser facilities.)

Product branding is when an organization operates a series of brands that are not supported by the corporate brand. The most famous example of this strategy is Procter & Gamble, which markets dozens of products as individual brands, including Tide and Ivory, with little or no connection to the Procter & Gamble name. Examples of product branding in healthcare abound, though often they are unintentional and inconsistent.

Hospitals often take a product branding approach with one or more specific service lines, specialty clinics, or centers. And at times, this approach is taken at the hospital level as well, such as with Partners Healthcare in Boston. Partners has many member hospitals, including Massachusetts General Hospital and Brigham and Women's Hospital.

There are pros and cons for each brand hierarchy strategy, though the most beneficial for health systems is usually unified branding (if it can be leveraged). The brand hierarchy strategy for your organization impacts many aspects of branding. For example, if your organization follows a product branding strategy, one entity may have a terrific brand in the market, but your other entities won't enjoy the halo effect afforded through a unified branding strategy.

Clearing the confusion

For a branding strategy to succeed, it is essential to start with an accurate understanding of what a brand is. In Chapter 3, we defined brand, branding, and key components of branding. But because the idea of branding is still relatively new in the healthcare provider industry, a lot of confusion exists between branding and other related concepts. In this chapter, we'll look at some of the common confusions and articulate how branding is related to each.

Branding versus marketing

More than any other word, *marketing* is most commonly confused with *branding*. This is perhaps understandable, given that the two are so similar in nature, scope, and intent. In fact, some experts don't even try to separate the two disciplines and just lump them together. In his book, *The 22 Immutable Laws of Branding*, Al Ries, one of the leading thinkers in the area of brand, says that "marketing is brand building. The two concepts are so inextricably linked that it's impossible to separate them. Furthermore, since everything a company does can contribute to the brand-building process, marketing is not a function that can be considered in isolation."

Whether it's "impossible" to separate the two, we'll soon argue. But on his last point, Ries is dead on: Marketing and branding cannot be considered in isolation from one another.

So, how are they different? Let's look at definitions again. We've already laid out a definition for branding—when an organization goes about trying to influence how audiences value the organization, its product, or its service. Philip Kotler is a leading marketing expert, and in his book, *Kotler on Marketing*, he defines *marketing* as "the art of finding, keeping, and growing profitable customers."

Does that make things clearer? Well, in some ways it does. For example, if we use Kotler's definition, branding is one strategy for pursuing marketing goals. Influencing how consumers value your organization will certainly make it easier to find, keep, and grow them as customers. Of course, there are other means for achieving marketing goals that don't fit the definition of branding. For example, offering a discount for patients to come in for a heart disease screening meets the goal of marketing, but not the goal of branding. This tactic will certainly influence the brand a consumer holds for your organization, but your intent is not merely to influence how consumers value your organization. Your intent is to persuade them to take action, try your service, and hopefully turn into profitable customers.

The idea of an action step can be useful in helping to distinguish between marketing efforts and branding efforts. Nearly all marketing efforts should have clear action steps, meaning that you want the recipient of the effort to do something. With branding, your intent isn't necessarily to have a consumer take action or do something, but rather to think or feel something. If you're successful in your branding effort, it will make it easier for consumers to act the way you desire when they next encounter your marketing efforts. As noted earlier, thousands of touch points influence brand, and the vast majority of these would not be considered to fall within the realm of marketing.

Another way to distinguish branding from marketing is to consider the time frames for each. Most marketing experts recommend marketing plans that extend no more than one or two years. Why? Because in that time frame, the market itself will have changed enough that many of the strategies and tactics in the plan will prove ineffective, and new opportunities and threats might be missed as well. In contrast, a brand strategy should be thought of not in years, but in decades. Building brands creates true transformation for an organization. It can take years to plan and implement brand-building strategies, and even longer to measure the impact of those strategies. From this perspective, marketing should be subservient to the brand strategy, with marketing strategies and tactics changing frequently but always supporting the overarching brand strategy.

In the end, the challenge is less about separating the definitions or intent of marketing or branding efforts, and more about ensuring that the two are always complementary to each other.

Branding versus mission

How is a brand strategy different from an organization's mission? A mission is usually described as a broadly framed statement of an organization's intent. Mission provides the answer to the question "What does the organization do?" For example, here is the mission statement for Rush University Medical Center in Chicago, posted on its Web site:

The Mission of Rush University Medical Center is to provide the very best care for our patients. Our education and research endeavors, community service programs and relationships with other hospitals are dedicated to enhancing excellence in patient care for the diverse communities of the Chicago area, now and in the future.

Of course, there are many varieties of mission statements, and their intent, use, and value vary among organizations. Although it's important for consumers to understand a healthcare provider's mission as part of the brand value they hold, it's rarely enough to build a strong brand. Knowing that a hospital treats patients in a given geographic area helps to lay the groundwork, but it isn't enough for a consumer to value that organization, assuming that other organizations with similar missions are vying for the consumer's attention. (In Chapter 6, we will look at the critical role that mission plays in distinguishing branding in healthcare from many other industries.)

Branding versus vision

Like a mission, a vision is a high-level statement intended to help guide an organization. Whereas a mission helps to articulate the basic "what" of an organization, a vision articulates the "why." More specifically, a vision captures the aspiration of where an organization wants to go, what it strives to achieve. Going back to Rush University Medical Center, here is its vision statement:

> *Rush University Medical Center will be recognized as the medical center of choice in the Chicago area and among the very best clinical centers in the United States.*

A vision statement is much closer in nature to a brand promise than a mission statement, as a vision often articulates a demonstrable and often differentiating value to consumers. I know from Rush's mission statement that it provides patient care for diverse communities in the Chicago area, but that's not enough for me to select its offerings over its competitors'. However, if I knew its vision and believed it was demonstrating that vision, now I have some clear reasons for choosing Rush over others: It is recognized as the medical center of choice in Chicago, and is among the very best clinical centers in the United States.

The key difference between an organization's vision and its brand strategy is that in most cases, the vision is intended to provide direction to internal audiences in what the organization hopes to achieve. A brand strategy articulates how the organization wants external audiences to value the organization. Sometimes an organization's vision can serve as its primary brand promise. But a brand promise doesn't have to mirror the vision, and at times it shouldn't.

For example, Rush could strive to achieve a recognized brand as the most technologically advanced provider of healthcare in the market.

Most experts would agree that an organization should understand and articulate its mission and vision before developing a brand strategy (though this isn't always the case). As with marketing and mission, the key with vision in relation to branding is that the two aren't necessarily the same, but that they must work congruently to move an organization forward.

Branding versus strategic planning

If a mission is the "what" and a vision is the "why," strategic planning is the "how." How will an organization deliver on its mission and move toward its vision? Of course, strategy can stand for many things in healthcare. There are marketing strategies, physician recruitment strategies, IT strategies, reimbursement strategies, and of course, brand strategies. Business guru Michael Porter helped to define strategy in a broad sense with his 1980 book, *Competitive Strategy*, in which he labels "generic strategies" as core ideas about how a firm can best compete in the marketplace. Porter lists only three potential generic strategies: low-cost leadership, differentiation of products or services, and a focus on a specific group of customers. Most organizations, however, don't restrict themselves to this definition.

Simply put, strategy is a plan for getting from point A to point B. At its highest level, strategic planning is the exercise of planning how an organization will achieve its long-term goals, usually looking at a horizon of three to five years.

Where branding is aimed at influencing how outside audiences value the organization, strategy is the means for delivering that value. Often, the elements of a strategic plan can have a profound impact on an organization's brand, but not always. For example, one of the most important strategies for healthcare providers is to improve safety within their organization, such as reducing medical errors or cutting the rate of postoperative infection. Although this might represent a key component of a hospital's strategic plan, a safety strategy does little in the way of building brand value. Why? Recall that a brand is the value, the emotion, the reputation a consumer gives any organization, product, or service. For the most part, consumers assume that the care they're receiving is safe. (The reality, of course, is often scarily different from this perception.) Trying to build a differentiated brand value around safety would most likely fail, as consumers already assume that the care you are offering is safe.

Consider the airline industry, where safety is just as strategic and crucial to success as it is in the healthcare provider world. Imagine an airline that tried to build its brand on being the "safest airline in the world." That would lead a consumer to infer that other airlines are less safe—yikes! The reality, of course, is that the level of safety varies among providers, and as a strategy, improving safety is crucial to the success of a healthcare provider, but most likely not in a brand-related way. This is not to say that safety can't have an impact on a provider's brand. Quite the contrary, a hospital with a poor track record of safety, or even with one well-publicized adverse event, will experience significant damage to its brand.

As with the other examples in this chapter, the key to separating organizational strategy from branding is to understand how they can support one another and to ensure that a high-level strategy doesn't run counter to an organization's desired brand. For example, it wouldn't make sense for a hospital that seeks to build a brand as offering the most qualified, experienced clinicians to institute a human resources strategy for only paying in the bottom quartile of physician salaries.

Branding versus positioning

Positioning is another business strategy that's closely related to branding. Whereas branding seeks to influence the value a consumer holds for an organization, positioning strives for the same result by trying to clearly position an organization in the consumer's mind relative to other options. The idea of positioning was first postulated by Al Ries and Jack Trout, pioneers in the use of branding in modern advertising and marketing. The idea behind positioning is that consumers are bombarded with thousands of messages every day, from hundreds of business categories and industries and thousands of products and services. There's no way to process it all, so consumers subconsciously filter and prioritize those brands that they trust, those that are familiar, and those that are prevalent. As Jack Trout writes in his book, *The Power of Simplicity*: "It must be simple, because minds hate complexity."

Often, brand strategy is driven by a positioning strategy. For example, the Domino's Pizza brand was built on a position based on fast delivery (as opposed to a position based on the quality or taste of the pizza). Volvo is known as the safe automotive choice (as opposed to the most stylish or least expensive). Establishing a clear, differentiated position in a market can be a huge competitive advantage for a company, because it makes brand-building and marketing efforts so much easier and less expensive.

However, given the nature of most healthcare provider organizations, it can be extraordinarily difficult to establish a truly differentiated position in a market. Most hospitals and health systems provide too many types of services to be known only for one, though there are exceptions (e.g., M.D. Anderson for cancer care). A great example of healthcare providers that own powerful positions are pediatric hospitals, where they often own the position of "best care for children" in their markets thanks in large part to their singular focus. Keep in mind that brand value comes both from the perception in the market that a focus in pediatrics must make that hospital better, and from the embodiment of that position, as their ability to focus decisions, resources, and more usually leads to an actual superior level of care.

Branding versus advertising

Brand leaders are often frustrated by those who equate advertising and branding. Many in healthcare—often physicians, but sometimes operational leaders—don't really understand the difference. For example, I heard a chief medical officer lament the large advertising expenditures the organization had made over the previous two years, which resulted in no change in market share. "Doesn't that prove that marketing doesn't work in healthcare?" he asked.

Advertising is a marketing tactic focused on external communication, and as I noted before, communications is one aspect of branding, but not the only aspect. Advertising's primary role in branding is to help raise awareness of a brand and articulate its key components to external audiences. This is done through paid placement of messages. Because the message is purchased space, the advertiser has complete control over its content and timing. However, because of its paid nature, advertising can lack the credibility of public relations, which raises awareness and communicates value by messages carried through unpaid third-party resources such as newspapers and magazines. Unlike advertising, there is no guarantee that a company will be "placed" or covered by the media. If successful, there is also no control over the content, tone, or timing.

Advertising and public relations can definitely support a branding effort in "telling a story," but first, as I've stressed, there must be a story to tell. Using puffery or weak claims does little to truly build brand in the market, and can often cause more damage than good.

Understanding advertising's role in building brand is also important from the perspective of managing internal expectations. Often, senior leaders will call for a brand advertising campaign, with the goal of increasing patient volumes. If it's truly a brand advertising campaign, it can help to increase volumes, but not in the way many people think. A brand advertising campaign seeks to raise awareness and communicate value using a long-term focus, hoping to build "mindshare" among potential consumers. Over hundreds or thousands of exposures, consumers will remember and value a particular brand without even having experienced it. Then, when they are compelled to act, either through their own needs or through a more focused marketing effort, they may seek out that organization. But this can take months, and more likely years, to have an effect. If leaders want increased surgical volumes next month, a brand advertising campaign will have minimal impact. More focused marketing strategies, such as offering community seminars or making outreach calls to key referring physicians, will more likely have a short-term impact (with advertising as a communications tactic supporting those efforts).

Reference

Pearce, John A., and Richard Robinson. *Formulation, Implementation, and Control of Competitive Strategy* (McGraw-Hill Companies: 2005), p. 23.

Branding myths

We've covered some of the common confusions related to branding, but some popular myths related to branding have also taken hold in healthcare. Some are related to this industry, but others are common throughout business. In either case, it's important to understand these myths so that they can be managed in your organization when building brands.

Myth #1: Branding doesn't matter in healthcare

Let's knock out the easiest myth first. This book provides ample evidence that branding matters in healthcare, as do the myriad other books, articles, and anecdotal stories from the field. However, those leading branding efforts will still encounter others who believe this. Thankfully, fewer and fewer CEOs and administrators are among those who cling to this myth. Most likely, they have read enough literature and seen enough other leaders—from inside and outside the healthcare industry—talk about the value of a strategic brand strategy that they would be unlikely to dismiss it outright.

Usually, this contention will come from others in administration, perhaps from the finance or human resources department, but most often it will be physicians who pooh-pooh the power of branding in healthcare. This may be somewhat understandable, as in many ways, branding lends value to all the elements of healthcare, not just the physician. Some docs get this idea and others find it offensive. As healthcare leaders, more and more physicians are also coming to realize that branding has a place at the table (even if they don't like it).

Those who don't believe that branding matters may point to the still-critical importance that proximity plays in where a patient goes: "People will go to the closest hospital—that hasn't changed." Another argument is that consumer decisions remain primarily influenced by physician referrals, which in many cases is still true. Or, the gatekeeping role of managed care will be raised.

Certainly, managed care influences consumer healthcare decisions. But in most cases, choice still exists for consumers within their plan. Proximity also plays a role in consumer decisions. However, any hospital or clinic that counts on proximity as its primary business driver is just asking for a competitor to come along and steal away its customers. How many competitors do you have within 20 miles?

The role that physicians play in guiding patients through direct referrals is still one of the primary channels for hospitals and health systems. That doesn't diminish the importance of branding, however. More and more, particularly with younger generations, patients are taking their physicians' referrals at face value and will continue to seek out other sources of information for making their healthcare decisions.

Finally, there's the clinical argument: "All that matters is the clinical outcome—the rest is window dressing." (Often, "clinical outcome" is replaced in this sentence by "physician's expertise" or "physician's experience.")

Positive clinical outcomes are essential to the success of a healthcare provider. But although clinical excellence is an important aspect of the value equation, in many cases it's no more important than experience, access, service, and price. In addition, these factors will increase in importance as consumers continue to spend more of their own money and enjoy more healthcare choices. In many markets, clinical excellence is often a commodity, and consumers assume a certain level of clinical excellence from their providers. It also can be extraordinarily difficult to measure, compare, or even find quality information on clinical quality, and it is difficult for consumers to evaluate what they do not understand. For all these reasons, focusing a provider brand on clinical excellence to the exclusion of the other elements of brand value may not be enough today. Unless the clinical product is demonstrably superior to the competition, clinical excellence just gets an organization on the playing field, it doesn't win the game.

At the risk of beating a dead horse, these times they are a changin'. Wherever consumers have choices, branding plays a role, and that most definitely is the world we face today in providing healthcare.

Myth #2: All hospitals are basically the same

The idea that you can't build a brand when you are not so different from all of your competitors is a tough one to dispell. There is some general truth to the myth that all hospitals are basically the same. Look around your market, whether it's a larger metropolitan area with a dozen hospitals or a rural setting where the closest hospital is 40 miles away. Most hospitals have an emergency room, maternity services, one large hospital building with a number of smaller ancillary buildings, and so on. Most pull from the same pool of physicians, and often, thanks to the industry's nursing shortage, most employ the same pool of nurses. Their missions are virtually the same, the strategies they employ are the same. Often, even their advertising looks the same.

Some of this is unavoidable, thanks to healthcare regulations, the responsibilities of community hospitals to provide emergent care, and so on. Most hospitals and health systems don't have the ability to focus exclusively on any one niche market, such as upper-income consumers or healthcare for those wanting the fastest service, as other businesses in other industries can pursue.

However, to claim that most hospitals in any given market are the same is clearly missing the reality of the situation. Organizations, like consumers, are individuals, with individual histories, cultures, strengths, and weaknesses. It may be hard to support a unique position in a market (using our definition from Chapter 4), but each hospital or health system most definitely has a unique brand and is served by distinguishing its brand as much as possible from other choices in the market, whether they are hospitals, free-standing surgical centers, mini clinics, or other providers.

Myth #3: Branding is dead

The myth that "Branding is dead" first started to appear after the Internet boom of the mid- to late 1990s, and it applied to the very concept of brands, not just healthcare brands. A November 2004 article in *Wired* magazine, "The Decline of Brands," argued that "sense of production is eroding in industry after industry, and instead of a consumer economy in which success is determined in large part by name, it's now being determined by performance. The aristocracy of brand is dead. Long live the meritocracy of product."

With access to more and more information, the argument goes, consumers are able to see through the "spin" of brandmiesters and view products and services for what they really are. They can make value judgments based on the "truth," not on "branding," through research on the Internet, the ability to share stories with other consumers through blogs or social networking, and more. The Internet was to usher in an era of transparency and "democracy" for consumers, allowing them to make rational decisions and diluting or eliminating the power of "brands."

The Internet did usher in an era of openness and transparency, but the value of brands didn't lessen. That's because with access to information on dozens or hundreds of options (think of online banking or buying a book), it was impossible for the average consumer to properly evaluate and keep track of all of his or her choices. Again, this is where brand is important. If you could order a computer from 1,000 different online retailers, where would you turn first? Most likely, you would turn to a retailer you knew and for which you had a positive perception. So, instead of making brands obsolete, the openness of the Internet in many ways made brands even more valuable.

Consider transparency in healthcare, related to the push to make pricing more accessible to consumers (another outcome of consumer-driven healthcare), or the publishing of more and more clinical quality data. Some would argue that transparency would lessen the value of branding in healthcare: If consumers can see the prices and the quality data, that's all that would matter, right? Again, simply providing data assumes that consumers make rational, objective decisions, which I showed in Chapter 1 is rarely the case (remember the Pepsi Challenge). If consumers were rational beings, the automobile quality and safety ratings in *Consumer Reports* would mirror consumer sales, yet millions of people still purchase fast cars, or cool cars, or expensive cars, and branding is a big reason why.

Myth #4: Brand-building is a short-term investment

Rarely is this actually articulated by a leader in a healthcare organization, but more often the myth that "Brand-building is a short-term investment" is demonstrated through the expectations or actions of healthcare leaders. For example, a leader may expect brand-building efforts to start in the first quarter, be completed in the second quarter, and show results by the fourth quarter: "This year, we'll focus on building our brands so that next year we can leverage our brand to do X, Y, or Z."

As most marketing leaders already know, brand-building is not measured in months or quarters, but years. As I've noted previously, it can take years simply to develop and employ a brand strategy, let alone for the strategy to take hold and show results. Sometimes this can be a difficult message to deliver to leaders, or others in the organization who need to buy into a branding effort. But the sooner the expectations of "immediate returns" are managed, the better for everyone involved.

Myth #5: Branding is the marketing department's job

The myth that "Branding is the marketing department's job" exists for a couple of key reasons. First, it comes from a confusion about what branding really is: "It's the logo" or "it's advertising." Because these elements emanate from the marketing department, branding must be the marketing department's job. As I showed in Chapter 4, these two elements are only part of the brand-building mix.

Second, much of brand-building typically does fall to the marketing leader. In most cases, the marketing leader in a healthcare organization will also be the primary driver of brand-building, leading the effort to develop a brand strategy, championing efforts to improve the brand experience, and of course, directing corporate identity projects, advertising campaigns, and other communication elements of branding.

However, given my definition in Chapter 3, brands are built from all touch points within an organization. From that standpoint, everyone is responsible for building brands, from the ICU charge nurse to the night-shift janitor to the star orthopedic surgeon. In addition, the role of organizational brand champion is best filled not by a marketing leader, but by the CEO or top administrator. As we'll see later, it's critical to have the top leader in the organization play a primary role in brand-building to ensure success.

Which of these myths are at play in your organization? Before embarking on a brand-building strategy, it's important to understand how those in your organization understand branding, and whether any of these, or other myths, have taken hold. You'll need to set the record straight to ensure a smooth brand-building process.

Branding is different in healthcare

Up to this point in the book, I've tried to paint a picture of branding as a business strategy that has as much value for a clinic or hospital as it does for an automaker or coffee shop. However, although I believe that branding holds the same potential value for healthcare providers as it does for other organizations, certain aspects of the healthcare industry make brand-building different for providers. Understanding these differences will help you to build a more successful brand.

Healthcare providers lack branding experience

As I noted in Chapter 2, branding as a strategy is relatively new to the world of healthcare providers. This impacts those trying to build brands in healthcare provider organizations in a number of ways.

First, there's an inherent learning curve with any brand-building effort. Hopefully, leadership will understand and value brands, though this should never be assumed. It's more likely that those who are responsible for building brands will need to spend more time than their brethren in other industries educating the next line of management in the organization—directors and managers—on the value of branding. Time and energy will also have to be spent with clinical leaders and physicians, as well as nurse managers, clinic managers, and more. This doesn't mean that branding can't be successful or that it shouldn't be attempted. It just means that leaders must have patience with brand-building efforts, should factor in the necessary education and training, and should assume a higher level of pushback than they might expect in other industries.

Second, because of branding's relative newness in the industry, it's difficult to find ample resources to support brand-building efforts. For example, case studies that show how a provider organization developed and implemented a brand strategy leading to demonstrable, long-term success are rare simply because it takes years to demonstrate that success. And at this time, the number of healthcare organizations that have even taken branding to a strategic, organization-wide level is low.

All of this means that branding has yet to hit a "critical mass" in healthcare, which can make it more difficult to successfully pursue. On the flip side, of course, those that can take the lead by leveraging brand-building should have a tremendous advantage compared with their competitors.

Limited pricing strategies limit brand options

In most other industries, companies can choose to compete in any number of aspects related to price alone. Take clothing retailers, where Kohl's has built its department store brand in large part on selling well-known clothing brands at low prices, whereas Nieman Marcus sells only the highest-priced clothing brands, yet both are successful companies. In technology, consumers can drop hundreds of dollars on a high-end iPhone from Apple, or get a phone for free as part of their calling plan from a cellular carrier.

For the most part, healthcare providers don't have the choice of differentiating their brand on price, either low or high. On the low side, certain built-in economic factors prevent lowering prices to compete effectively, most importantly from a cost-of-labor perspective. A limited labor pool of physicians and nurses means that costs for this primary expense will always remain relatively high (though it remains to be seen what impact globalization will have on labor costs). Perhaps more important, it wouldn't be smart to pin a brand differentiation on low price in healthcare. In some areas, certainly, low price can be a competitive benefit (e.g., prescription drugs and vaccinations), and providers will eventually need to be competitive pricewise on nearly any service they offer. Research shows that roughly 10% of all consumers are driven primarily by price alone.

But few consumers are likely to equate "lowest price" in healthcare with the best choice for their healthcare needs. After all, in many cases, healthcare is a matter of life and death, or more often, a comfortable, pain-free life. "Lowest price" often equates to "lowest quality," something most consumers would conceivably not be willing to accept when it comes to their own health or that of their loved ones.

On the high side, a number of market and regulatory forces restrict healthcare providers from pricing services higher, even for services that provide more value. Prices are often set by negotiated contracts with payers, so even if a service could be valued at $5,000 and a consumer would be willing to pay that, if the contract says the billing should be $3,000, that's the billing. Medicare also limits what patients can be charged, and in the past has made rulings that even limit the ability of physicians, clinics, or hospitals to sell "added value" services such as concierge care or more personalized care from physicians. These restrictions, of course, vary from service to service, and many organizations that provide primarily cosmetic surgery, alternative medicine, or other elective procedures have more flexibility to use price to differentiate their brands. But for most hospitals and health systems, this value factor isn't an option.

Mission trumps brand every time

In many industries, brand-building can supercede the actual product or service being provided. An organization that considers itself "brand-driven" pays as much attention—or more—to the holistic strategy of building its brand as it does the product or service the brand initially supported. In these types of organizations, the brand strategy may well determine what products are launched next, rather than the products driving the brand.

For example, take Starbucks, where the drive to create an experiential brand based on environment, service, music, and more has as much or greater impact than the product itself, the coffee. Or Apple, which considers its brand differentiation tied to "innovative design," a brand promise that allows it to move from producing computers to developing the iPod, while still staying true to its brand. Or UPS, which broadened its brand beyond simply shipping packages to providing complete supply-chain management and strategies for its clients.

For healthcare providers—specifically clinics, hospitals, and health systems—their mission of offering services tied to the care of patients will always be first and foremost. No matter the provider organization and no matter the brand strategy pursued, the core players (physicians, nurses, etc.) will show up in a similar way—delivering on the mission of providing great care to patients.

Again, this isn't to say that branding doesn't have value, or to support the myth that "All providers are the same." Instead, it acknowledges the rightful place clinical care has in the hierarchy of responsibilities for physicians, nurses, and all other staff members in a healthcare provider organization. In some organizations, staff members might be particularly friendly, lending to brand differentiation. Or the staff might have a higher level of clinical expertise, lending to brand differentiation. Or an organization may use the latest technologies, or deliver more personalized care, or whatever else lends itself to brand differentiation. In each case, the organization is building a differentiated brand, but in each case, when it comes down to the actual interaction between the customer and the organization, the mission of delivering care takes precedence. The brand-building aspect is, at worst, second on the list. At best, it's interwoven directly into the care. But the reason that nurse does her job hasn't—and won't—change. Brand supplements the mission, enhances the mission, even differentiates the mission, but it can't supercede the mission.

As you'll see later in the book, acknowledging this reality relieves some of the brand-building pressures that leaders might feel and allows for more realistic brand-building efforts.

Developing a brand strategy

Once you've decided to actively build and manage your brand, the next step is to create a brand strategy. As described in Chapter 3, a brand strategy is a guiding blueprint for how an organization wants to brand itself for the future. A brand strategy might also be called a brand map, a brand plan, or any number of other similar names, but the idea is the same: the expression of the key components of an organization's desired brand.

Six steps to developing your brand strategy

In this chapter, we'll walk through a six-step process for developing a brand strategy. There are as many approaches to developing a brand strategy as there are books on branding. Some are more complicated, others simpler. Some rely heavily on a consultant's proprietary model or perspective whereas others take a more open, formative approach. The process you use will most likely depend on the firm or individual you hire to help you with the process. Most follow a standard path, with the same key steps outlined here.

When considering hiring outside help, use this outline as a guide. Where you find variances, ask questions about what might be missing, or the value of added steps or exercises. There is no right or wrong process, and each branding expert has developed one that is comfortable for him or her. The key is to make sure you are comfortable with the process and that you understand exactly what it entails.

No matter what path you take, your destination in this process is a brand strategy that captures the high-level elements that define your brand. Usually, the brand strategy is expressed in a written document, but there are other ways you can capture the elements of your brand strategy, as we'll see later.

Step 1: Identify internal participants

For a brand strategy to have any hope for success, it must be developed using the input of organizational leaders. One of the best ways to sentence a brand strategy to the graveyard of lost initiatives is to have a marketing or other executive develop the brand strategy and then take it to leadership for approval. Without having invested the time, energy, and pain of thinking through the critical aspects of branding, it's virtually impossible to expect organizational leaders to own the brand strategy (though as we will see in our case studies, there's always an exception to the rule). Without that ownership, most leaders will be hard-pressed to support branding efforts on a long-term basis. Truly living a brand requires discipline, constant communication, and hard decisions from leaders. Without ownership, it's too easy to avoid those difficult challenges, dooming branding efforts to failure.

In fact, the best-case scenario is to have the CEO or administrator initiate development of a brand strategy. This guarantees ownership right from the start. For some lucky organizations, this comes naturally. Maybe the top executive learns from a peer about the value of branding, or attends a conference and "gets branding religion." Or maybe a new CEO comes on board and brings with him or her a passion for branding. Although these situations do occur occasionally in healthcare, they are rarer in this industry than in others because most leaders of provider organizations rise up through similar paths. Top leaders often come from operations or finance, or are physicians— none of which typically provides significant exposure to branding.

If a CEO or administrator isn't driving the brand strategy initially, it's usually up to the top marketing executive to make branding a priority. This can be triggered in a number of ways. Sometimes a dramatic event in the market can drive new thinking, such as a competitor opening a new surgical center or announcing a multimillion-dollar renovation. Or perhaps long-simmering trends, such as declining market share or weakening patient satisfaction surveys, can be turned into a "burning platform" to drive change. Another, subtler approach would be to slowly expose a leader to branding as a strategy, and let the CEO "discover" its value him or herself. You can do this by referring the leader to articles or books, having the leader attend sessions on branding at conferences, raising the topic at high-level meetings, and so on.

No matter how you do it, your organization's top leader must be on board with the development of brand strategy before the process begins. From there, the next step is to develop a brand strategy steering committee to participate in the development process. In addition to the CEO or administrator, other key participants should include:

- COO, if separate from top administrator
- CFO or top financial executive
- CNO or top patient care executive
- CIO or top technology officer
- CMO or top physician executive
- Top human resources executive
- Top marketing/new business development executive

These executives are critical to include in the process, given their leadership in core functional areas. You also may want to include leaders from other organizational functions, such as facilities, quality and safety, or organizational development. Or you may want to include the directors of top service lines or administrators of individual facilities. Some organizations invite the entire leadership group, which can include top executives and all directors. Depending on the organization, this could become unwieldy: It's difficult to get a group of 100 to agree on anything. The best size of group for this type of collaborative process is usually six to 12 people, but including the right people is more important than focusing on a certain quantity. Your branding consultant should have recommendations regarding the group's size and composition.

Typically, the top marketing executive manages the brand strategy development process. Although others in the organization can drive this process, it's critical that the process owner fundamentally understands and values branding. It's too much to ask the process owner to learn on the job with such an often-misunderstood concept as branding. Later, we'll talk about individual roles that are necessary when making the brand strategy come to life.

SHOULD PHYSICIANS PARTICIPATE IN THE DEVELOPMENT OF THE BRAND STRATEGY?

You may be wondering whether physicians should participate in the development of the brand strategy. The answer here is a resounding "yes". Often, executives make the mistake of not including top physicians in the process. Sometimes they assume that physicians won't have the time to participate or don't want to be bothered with branding. Other times, leaders don't want to invite the political challenges that come with including some physicians but not others. Whatever the reason, not including top physicians is a mistake. First, physicians are the foundation of patients' brand experience, and they often have the greatest ability to make an impact on patients at an individual level. Second, although it's frequently difficult to differentiate a provider's brand based on clinical care, it is obviously the core service of a healthcare provider organization, and physicians are the leaders in shaping that delivery. Third, physicians often don't understand or value branding, which makes it difficult to convince them to embrace brand-building. Having physicians involved in the brand's strategic development will help to bridge that gap, making it easier for doctors throughout the organization to buy into the brand strategy.

At a minimum, organizations should include a top physician executive, such as a CMO or vice president of medical affairs. Other influential physicians could be considered, such as a top surgeon or a physician who's long been active in the organization. These may be independent physicians, not employed by the hospital or health system. In these cases, it's important to consider potential competitive conflicts of interest, such as whether a key referring physician also rounds at a competing hospital.

Step 2: Identify an external partner

Most organizations will engage an external partner to drive the brand strategy development process. Although this is not an absolute requirement—anyone with experience in brand-building could lead the process—it's highly recommended for a number of reasons.

First, an external brand consultant will bring focused energy to the process. Given all the day-to-day activities for which a senior marketing executive is responsible, it would be difficult to carve out the time and energy needed to lead such an intensive process. Marketing executives may assume that they can save funds by keeping the process in-house. Or they may feel they have enough experience to lead the process themselves (which some do). But inevitably, when the next big crisis hits, the brand strategy process will get delayed, or everyday pressures will stretch the process beyond the intended schedule. Keeping the process moving and keeping participants focused is important to a successful outcome, and an external consultant can help to ensure that this happens.

Second, an external consultant will bring the aura of expertise to the table, which, like it or not, is crucial to the process. Top marketing executives often lament the "deaf ears" effect, which describes what they encounter when stressing an important issue such as branding, only to have an outside consultant come in and preach the same message with much greater success. "What is the importance of the patient experience to our brand? I've been saying that for years," they say. "Now, in one meeting, the consultant has everyone nodding his head and saying, 'Wow, patient experience is really important.' "

Although understandably frustrating, this phenomenon is fairly typical in any large organization. Leaders often give credence to the word of an outside consultant over their own executives, even when the message is the same. Instead of fighting this effect, savvy marketing leaders leverage it to ensure that important aspects of branding are driven home by their external partners. An external consultant also can make the process smoother because organizational participants are less likely to question a basic idea or philosophy, which happens with those unfamiliar with a concept. A physician is less likely to question the value of the patient experience if it's extolled by an expert than if it is pushed by an executive within the organization.

Third, a brand consultant will offer a proven process, which is absolutely critical to emerging from the effort with a solid brand strategy. Discussing brand elements such as values and promises is notoriously subjective and doesn't lend itself to the clear, left-brain thinking many executives and physicians prefer. For that reason, the branding discussions may go far a field, and dialogue can become deeply esoteric—all of which is fine, but requires an experienced facilitator working within a known structure to avoid driving off the tracks. A proven brand process will account for—and even encourage—this type of broad, subjective thinking and will ensure a successful ending to the process. It will be important for the internal process owner, organizational leaders, and group participants to trust that if the group is off in left field, the external consultant can bring the group back on track.

Fourth, and perhaps most important, a branding consultant will bring an outside, objective viewpoint to the table. It is extraordinarily difficult for organizational executives to see the forest for the trees when it comes to branding and their market. They are just too close to the scene to be objective or to see potential opportunities from a customer's perspective. Because a brand consultant doesn't bring a personal history with the organization to the table, he or she will be able to see the obvious and can look at the situation with a new, unfiltered view, which is critical to developing a powerful brand strategy. In addition, an outside consultant is able to ask "stupid questions" without fear, questions that often challenge long-held beliefs or sacred cows. "You've always provided primary care with one physician group partner. Why is that?" He or she also should be able to challenge executives who try to force their opinions on the group without fear of reprisal, which can be difficult or impossible for an internal executive to pull off.

Who should you engage as your brand strategy partner? The options are unlimited, and they range from individual consultants to large branding firms or advertising agencies. Carefully consider whether you want an independent consultant or a firm as your partner. There are pros and cons of each. Some of the leading experts on brand are independent consultants, and they offer a greater ability to focus exclusively on your engagement. Firms or agencies can bring multiple experts with multiple perspectives to the process, and they have the support staff to help facilitate the process. In either case, the consultant must be able to manage research development as necessary (though keep in mind that he or she doesn't have to provide research services, as an outside research specialist can be engaged if necessary). In the end, the size of the consultant's business doesn't matter—the consultant's expertise and your personal comfort with him or her do.

The credentials of a partner firm are important, but the most important aspect is to understand exactly who will be leading the brand strategy process. You should expect an experienced brand expert, usually an independent consultant or a senior principal or partner at a firm. Regardless of the firm's experience, it's the experience of the lead consultant that matters. This person should know branding inside and out, should have experience leading brand strategy development efforts, and should be deft at working with senior leaders and physicians. Because it's difficult to judge these qualities from a Web site or interview, be sure to request referrals pertaining to the potential candidate. Better yet, ask your peers who've gone through the process which consultant they used and whether they would recommend the firm.

More than experience or process, the most important attribute of a brand consultant is whether his or her personality is the right fit for you and your organization. Some consultants are more laid back in their approach, letting the process evolve organically. Some consultants are more "Type A" and rigid in their approach to process. Some are aggressive and opinionated. Others are pure facilitators who let the internal team drive all opinions and decisions. In the best-case scenario, you want a partner who can bring all of these qualities to bear as necessary, avoiding "one-trick ponies."

Although there are differing opinions on the subject, I highly recommend engaging a partner experienced with branding in the healthcare provider sector. Brand strategy is a fundamental business strategy, so its development requires a fundamental understanding of the business of healthcare—the role of reimbursement to the business model, and the influence of Medicare and other insurance payers; the regulations and laws governing medical care, such as Stark laws and the Health Insurance Portability and Accountability Act of 1996; the unique influence physicians have in provider organizations; and the dynamics of hospital organizations. A brand consultant doesn't have to be an expert in all of these areas, but he or she must understand the business of providing healthcare, which is best gained from experience in working in the industry. A branding partner who confuses key business concepts, or misstates an obvious aspect of the business during the process, quickly loses credibility with participants, which can poison the entire initiative.

On the other hand, the healthcare provider industry is notoriously insular. Hospital executives almost universally come up through the ranks, rarely joining a hospital or system from outside the industry. Hospitals and health systems usually look first and foremost to their peers for ideas and benchmarking, rather than to other industries. All of this has been a leading reason why branding has been so late in coming to healthcare in the first place. Although it's important that your partner has experience in healthcare, it's also beneficial to find a partner who has experience in other fields as well. This allows them to bring a more holistic approach to the branding process, and to push the boundaries beyond traditional healthcare thinking.

When choosing a firm or agency, give special consideration to the business offerings of that firm. Make sure it can provide brand strategy guidance independent of other services, such as corporate identity design or advertising. Unfortunately, many traditional advertising agencies approach brand-building from an advertising perspective—as a vehicle to drive external promotions.

Although it does serve that purpose, as we've discussed, a brand strategy must first address how an organization lives its brand, from which external communication flows, not the other way around. Avoid firms that use a brand strategy process as simply a precursor to developing an advertising campaign. In the same vein, avoid design firms that are driven by the opportunity to redesign the corporate identity. Although a new name or corporate identity may result from a brand-building process, it shouldn't be the driving factor behind one. If a consultant is recommending a new name for the organization, you want to know that it's because that recommendation is in your best interest, not theirs.

That doesn't mean you should avoid any firm that creates advertising or designs corporate identities. On the contrary, a partner with these services can prove useful down the road if advertising or corporate identity work is required. Because it was involved in the development of your brand strategy, it should know the brand intimately, leading to easier and more successful communications or identity work. Pay attention to how a firm approaches brand strategy work: Can it focus exclusively on this work, without tying it to other services down the road? Does it have examples of other clients that have hired the firm for brand strategy alone? Do the firm's fees reflect an honest branding engagement, or are you receiving a discounted price in the hope that you'll buy more down the road? Again, the best approach is to ask around and see what your peers have to say about the firms you're considering.

Typically, the internal owner of the process will head the search for an outside partner with input from the CEO or a select few other leaders. Once a partner is chosen, an agreement should be signed that designates costs, specific process parameters, a schedule, and more. Some of the details can be worked out after the consultant is hired, such as specific meeting dates or optional elements of the process. The internal marketing lead will then work with the consultant to formalize key aspects of the process in preparation for the kickoff session.

Step 3: Hold a kickoff session

With the internal branding team and external brand partner in place, it's important to have a formal kickoff for the process. Typically, this occurs in a session led by the brand consultant, but it also can include communication leading up to the session or following it. For example, participants may be given homework to prepare for the process, which might include reading articles, books, or existing research, or performing activities to help engage the participants in branding. Or they may receive a questionnaire to help gauge their level of understanding of brand.

The actual kickoff session accomplishes a number of goals:

- It lets the participants meet the brand consultant in person for the first time (the marketing leader, and maybe even the CEO, will have met the consultant in the interview process)

- It allows the brand consultant to outline the process, reviewing the process steps, schedules, roles and responsibilities of participants, rules of engagement, and more

- It provides an opportunity for the CEO or administrator to communicate his or her commitment to the process

- It provides a forum for participants to ask questions about the process, or about branding itself

Many times, the kickoff meeting will include activities to help further engage the participants. No matter the structure, the kickoff meeting provides a formal initiation of the process, which helps to set the stage for the importance of the work.

Step 4: Gauge your current brand

A brand strategy is *aspirational*, providing guidance to where you want your brand to be in the future. Without knowing where you are today, however, it will be impossible to set a course for where to go tomorrow. Unless you're a start-up company, your organization already has an existing brand. So, before you begin to craft your brand strategy, it's critical to understand what your brand is today.

In measuring your current brand, you're evaluating how your organization is perceived and valued in the market you serve. This brand perception may be different from the reality of the situation. For example, your community may say they see you as a bare-bones cost-cutting corporation because 10 years ago you had significant layoffs. Though in reality this perception doesn't reflect the true nature of your financial actions today, it doesn't matter. With branding, perception is reality. Your goal is to understand current perceptions to align them with the brand you desire.

There are many ways to measure your current brand. In many cases, data will already exist, and you'll just need to collect and analyze it. But more likely, new research will be required. Your brand consultant partner should guide you in understanding what existing information is valuable and what information may be needed. If you need to gather new research, you may need to engage a research specialist, or your brand consultant may be able to provide research services.

Here are the typical sources for gauging your existing brand, along with some considerations. Although each lends unique value in understanding your brand, none is sufficient by itself for gaining a complete picture.

Community perception surveys

Community perception surveys go by different names, but in essence, these are surveys that hospitals and health systems conduct to see how they are perceived in a market. They ask consumers questions such as "Which hospital first comes to mind?" or "Where do you normally go for healthcare services?" These surveys provide a great benchmark for measuring awareness and perception over time and are great at identifying overriding differentiators, such as which hospital has the best reputation in a market for cardiac care. The downside of any survey is that it provides only surface-level feedback and doesn't allow a researcher to dive deep into the psyche of an individual to understand unconscious and emotional brand perceptions. In addition, surveys don't always attract a balanced sampling of a market, and consumers are apt to say one thing while doing something completely different. A survey may capture an individual's perceived beliefs at a moment in time, but those beliefs don't always correlate with how that individual will behave tomorrow. Most healthcare providers conduct community perception surveys on an ongoing basis. For survey results to be useful for a brand strategy process, they should be no more than two years old, and preferably as recent as the current year.

Patient satisfaction surveys

Another tool used today by nearly all healthcare providers in one form or another is the patient satisfaction survey, which provides a terrific benchmark for measuring your service levels over time. As surveys, though, they also have the same limitations as community perception surveys.

Employee satisfaction surveys

Employee satisfaction surveys provide valuable feedback on internal perceptions of the organization, with the same caveats regarding surveys as noted in the preceding two sections.

Community focus groups

Focus groups are great for hearing the voice of the customer firsthand, as well as demonstrating interest in the market's thoughts and opinions. Unfortunately, focus groups are easily misunderstood and misused in healthcare. Because there is a direct exposure to the "voice of the customer," the results can be given too much weight in judging consumer perceptions. The dangers of group dynamics are well documented, from the power of a particularly articulate or vocal member to bias group perceptions, to the potential for "group think." Although focus groups are a natural tool for helping to measure market feedback, they need to be well facilitated, and results must be considered as one part of the picture, not the entire picture.

One-on-one customer interviews

Another issue with focus groups is that, like surveys, they don't easily allow for the deeper exploration of an individual's unconscious thoughts, which is important for understanding brands. Individual interviews, however, do allow for such exploration. In a great book on the topic of consumer research, *How Customers Think: Essential Insights into the Mind of the Market*, Harvard Business School professor Gerald Zaltman uses research to show that 90% of what influences a consumer's decisions and preferences lies in the unconscious mind. Because surveys (and often focus groups) tap only the conscious mind, they miss true insights into the preferences of consumers. In fact, consumers are not aware of the hundreds or thousands of factors that influence their decisions and preferences, so simply asking for information in a survey will rarely expose the deeper insights necessary to make breakthroughs in understanding brand perceptions.

Zaltman's book proposes in-depth interviews using storytelling and metaphor as a better way to collect information from consumers. When conducting any type of interview, it's important to use an outside facilitator. In addition to bringing interview experience, an outside facilitator brings a level of safety to the setting, allowing an interviewee to feel more comfortable expressing honest, and sometimes emotional, thoughts. Again, the brand consultant or members of the firm's staff may be experienced in this area, or you can find an outside research partner to conduct the interviews.

Internal interviews

The same reasons for conducting one-on-one interviews with customers apply to internal audiences. To start, all members of the brand strategy process team should be interviewed. Not only do they have some of the best information on how the organization is perceived, but also it's important for the brand consultant to have "heard" all participants in the process. This gives all participants the opportunity to provide candid opinions without fear of reprisal. In addition to the branding team, interviews can be conducted with representatives from throughout the organization, whether they are physicians, nurses, managers, or staff members. It helps to get a broad sampling of the organization, and for those who have geographically diverse organizations, different areas and facilities should be represented.

There is a point of diminishing returns with internal interviews. Often, with one dozen to two dozen interviews, the broad themes and perceptions are captured and additional interviews will reveal little new information.

Editorial review

An editorial review involves the culling of all media coverage of the organization over time, going back usually two to five years, though the time frame can be longer. An editorial review allows the team to see how a key influencer—the media—perceives the organization. For example, does coverage over time tend to be more positive or more negative? Is there a certain specialty, such as trauma care or oncology, for which the media tends to turn to your organization (or to your competitors)?

In addition to traditional sources of coverage, such as newspapers, magazines, or television, an editorial review also should include ratings services, health information Web sites, and any other resource that provides public evaluation of the organization.

Understanding your current brand perception in the market is critical to the brand strategy process, but the research effort shouldn't overwhelm the process. Some of these tactics can take months to complete, and they may be vital to understanding the brand. But at some point, you need to feel that you have "enough" data to move forward. Your outside partner should be able to provide guidance as to when "enough is enough."

Once the research has been collected, the brand consultant should analyze it and feed it back to the group in a findings report. The findings report should include an executive summary and should highlight important points, but it also should include as much raw data as feasible. This allows those who desire to dig deeper the opportunity to do so, and helps to alleviate any potential concerns that the findings have been somehow manipulated to support a particular opinion or outcome. If all goes right, the findings report should not reveal too many big surprises. Hopefully, it's a reflection of what organizational leaders already know about how the organization is perceived in the market. But the findings report delivery is an opportunity to check in and ensure that everyone is on the same page regarding how the existing brand is perceived. If there are discrepancies, the process should allow for discussion of the differences, and the means to correct erroneous information, update current thinking, and in some cases, accept that different participants can agree to disagree on certain points so that the process can continue.

Step 5: Develop the core elements of the brand strategy

All of the effort to this point in the process is to prepare the group for the hard work of developing the core elements of the brand strategy. Before we explore how these elements are developed, let's take a deeper look at the three elements found in most every brand strategy.

As noted in Chapter 3, brand strategies typically contain at least three core elements, which are depicted in Figure 7.1, which helps to demonstrate their relevance to each other.

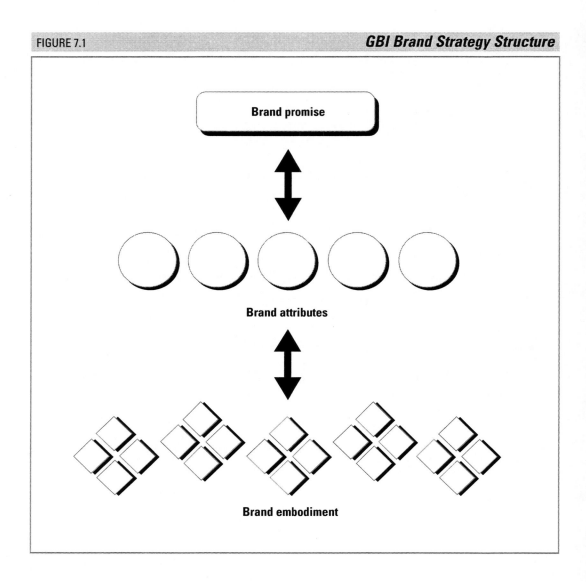

FIGURE 7.1　　　　　　　　　　　　　　　*GBI Brand Strategy Structure*

Brand promise

Brand attributes

Brand embodiment

The brand promise

Sometimes the brand promise is referred to as the brand positioning statement, or simply the positioning statement, or even the value proposition (though this latter term has a different meaning for many marketers). No matter the exact terminology, the brand promise is the overarching descriptor of the brand an organization wants its audiences to hold in their minds and hearts about it. If possible, it should be expressed in one phrase or sentence. Some organizations choose a longer brand promise, which might encompass a series of statements, or a set of core ideas regarding what the brand should represent. Either way, the purpose is to provide a simple, clear depiction of the desired brand. In essence, it represents the desired answer to this question posed to the typical consumer: "How do you feel about our organization?" In a perfect world, the majority of responses would mirror the brand promise.

Internally, the brand promise serves as a statement of how employees should aspire to show up every day, guiding actions, decisions, thoughts, and motivations. It should be grounded in today's truth, but more important, the brand promise should provide a direction for tomorrow. Although the brand promise is aspirational, it should not be expected that at some point the organization will ever fully reach the desired brand and branding efforts will come to an end. Branding is more about the journey, not the destination.

Brand attributes

Brand attributes are also often referred to as brand values, brand drivers, or brand descriptors. These represent the values or essence of the desired brand, and they should provide support for the brand promise. Brand attributes are most often framed in single words, such as *passionate* or *first-class*. Although there is no perfect number of brand attributes, the goal should be to limit these elements to no more than six, so they can truly serve as guiding priorities. These elements help to lend further definition to the brand promise, and they allow those in the organization easier access to understanding and living the brand. For example, whereas the brand promise provides a general, conceptual statement of the desired brand, the brand attributes provide actionable qualities from which the staff can take action.

In describing brand attributes, it often helps to use definitions, customer statements, and even visuals to clarify the concept. For example, if a brand attribute is "convenient," the brand strategy might go on to define "convenient" as "ease of obtaining care." First-person customer statements such as "I want your services to be close to my home" or "I want to have access to care at times that are convenient for me, such as on weekends" might be used to help clarify what "convenient" means to the market.

Brand embodiment

Whereas the brand promise and attributes are concepts that define the desired brand, brand embodiment points provide real-life examples of ways an organization demonstrates and communicates its brand. Brand embodiment is the proof that backs up the promise. Brand embodiment can take the form of patient stories, awards or recognition, research results, financial metrics, clinical outcomes, rankings, and more.

For example, using the "convenient" brand attribute, potential brand embodiment points might include:

- The addition of three new mini clinics by the organization in the previous year

- Better-than-average wait times in the ER

- A letter from a patient commending a physician for taking time after hours to speak about a health issue

When developing the brand strategy, it's important to have at least a few brand embodiment points to support each brand attribute. Depending on the existing brand perceptions and realities, however, some brand attributes may be more easily supported than others. For example, the organization may be ahead of the competition in providing convenient services, but needs some work on providing friendly service to support another brand attribute of "caring." Even for those attributes that need more work, it's still important to find at least a couple of brand embodiment points, as these real-life examples are tools that help the staff to understand the desired brand and give them ideas regarding how they can individually support the brand.

Developing the brand elements

Now that we have a better understanding of the elements found in a brand strategy, let's consider how these are developed. Again, there are many approaches to this step in the process. Each brand consultant will have his or her own means for working with an organization to create the brand elements. Following are some guidelines for this critical step in the brand strategy process.

The brand strategy model shown in Figure 7.1 shows the brand promise at the top of the chart, depicting its place as the ultimate expression of the desired brand. However, in the development of the brand strategy, it helps to start at the second level, with the identification and selection of the brand attributes. A laundry list of potential attributes will come naturally from the research, making this an easy starting point for discussion. This is an area where participants truly can contribute to the brand strategy with their own ideas. Although the brand consultant can provide an initial list of potential attributes, participants easily can add others of their own, or eliminate those they don't feel are as important. The list can then be pared down through any number of techniques (such as multi-voting or forced-choice ranking). Once the final attributes are chosen, it then becomes easier to have context for development of the brand promise.

Although development of the brand attributes can be a collaborative exercise, when it comes to the brand promise it's often better to have the consultant develop a number of alternatives to bring to the group for consideration. Whether there are six participants or 26, it can be nearly impossible for a group of any size to collaboratively construct something as concise and powerful as a brand promise statement. Instead, this is where the brand consultant can lend expertise in crafting a number of statements and helping the group evaluate the options. Often, the group will dissect one or more options, replacing words or whole ideas in the process. This should be expected, and even encouraged, but it is usually much less painful than having the group create a statement from scratch.

When evaluating the brand promise, consider using the following six criteria. The more a brand promise meets each criterion, the more successful your brand-building will be.

1. **Customer need:** How well does the brand promise address a core customer need? This may seem obvious, but some organizations get so wrapped up in what they want to accomplish that they forget it has to be something their customers will value. If your brand doesn't meet a core customer need, it's doomed to failure.

2. **Realness:** How well does your brand promise reflect reality? Again, a brand strategy is meant to be aspirational, providing a guiding vision for how your organization wants to be valued by the market moving forward. But it also must be grounded in reality. If you are a small community hospital and you seek to be valued as a top tertiary referral center in the region, how realistic is that goal? Will you be able to attract top specialists? Do you have the capital to make the necessary investments in technology? Remember, perhaps the most damaging move an organization can make relative to branding is to make a promise on which it can't deliver. If you can deliver on only 10% of the promise now, make sure your external communications reflect this reality.

As you develop the brand promise, the findings report that articulates how your brand is currently perceived should serve as a touch point. If you're happy with the current brand perception and you want a brand promise that reflects it, realness is less of an issue. However, if you're trying to build a brand promise that improves upon current market perceptions, make certain you can walk the walk.

3. **Believability:** Even if your brand promise is grounded in reality or could be potentially real, how believable is it? If you've never had a strong reputation as a cardiac center but your brand promise expresses a vision of being recognized as a top heart center in the country, will your market believe it? Even if you're committed to what it takes internally to make that brand promise a reality, carefully consider how easy it will be to persuade the market that you can deliver on the promise. As with realness, use the findings on your current brand perception as a guide. Just because your desired brand may not sound believable now, based on current market perceptions you shouldn't necessarily abandon the pursuit of a highly aspirational brand. But it will be important to honestly assess the additional energy and resources it may take to get you there.

4. **Sustainability:** How sustainable is your brand promise? First, will you be able to deliver your brand promise over a long period of time? Brand-building efforts can take years to implement and show results. Are you prepared to stick with the brand promise for that length of time? Second, how sustainable is the brand promise from a market perspective? That is, will the promise you're making still be valued or

relevant in five or 10 years, or have you chosen something so narrow or trendy that it could lose its impact down the road? Finally, will your brand promise allow you to sustain your organization financially over the coming years? For example, if you decide to make a promise for offering the most affordable care in the market, will you be able to generate enough income to invest in necessary improvements or survive market downturns?

5. **Focus:** How focused is your brand promise? This is where the traditional definition of positioning comes in. From Chapter 3, we learned that positioning is a strategy for trying to own a specific niche or value point in a market, such as Domino's with fast delivery or Volvo with safety. There are many advantages to a focused position, but as we also learned, it can be difficult for a traditional hospital or healthcare system to focus its brand so narrowly in the market. Too many aspects of care are delivered.

Although a healthcare provider might be challenged to narrow its brand relative to service offerings, it would be wise to consider how to focus its brand on how it offers its services. There's an old saying that if a company claims it offers the fastest, cheapest, and best service, odds are it delivers on none of those claims. That's because most of us, from experience, understand that it's virtually impossible to be the best at everything, and those who claim this test the limits of believability. If a hospital creates a brand promise that claims the organization offers the highest level of clinical expertise, with the most caring staff and the best patient experience, can they truly deliver all three? Of course, most healthcare organizations would strive to excel in these areas, and more.

Although the drive for focus should be taken seriously, it is often difficult to land on a brand promise that unites the organization on one key value, and brand strategy teams shouldn't become stuck trying to achieve this attribute.

6. **Uniqueness:** Is your brand promise unique? Again, like the attribute of focus, it can be hard for hospitals or health systems to be truly unique in a market. However, the whole intent of brand-building is to create differentiation from your competitors, and this differentiation can have its roots in the brand promise. However, differentiation in provider healthcare often comes not from the stated brand promise, but from how you deliver on that promise.

Step 6: Documenting the brand strategy

Once you've landed on the core elements, it's time to capture the brand strategy. Usually this is accomplished through the creation of a brand strategy document, or "brand book." The brand book is usually generated by the brand consultant and typically includes the following:

- An introductory letter from the CEO/administrator
- An overview of the brand-building process, including a list of participants
- An introduction to the meaning and value of brand

- A description of the core elements and their purpose
- A sampling of brand embodiment points
- Other elements as necessary

You should write the brand book so that anyone in the organization can read and understand it, regardless of his or her role or existing understanding of brand. In the next chapter, we'll look at how you can use the brand book to build the brand internally, as well as how other tools can capture and communicate the brand strategy.

Once the brand strategy is finalized and documented, some organizations will test their brand strategy and its elements with critical audiences, such as staff, physicians, or consumers. Be careful in how you conduct this testing. As I've noted, most internal audiences and consumers don't understand or value branding and will be hard-pressed to provide credible feedback on the worthiness of the brand elements you've selected. Rather than asking these audiences to judge the elements of your brand, you may find more value in asking for their interpretation of key elements. For example, asking a consumer "What does convenient mean to you?" may lead to insights in how best to deliver on that aspect of a brand promise.

In the end, you need to trust your organizational leaders and brand consultant partner to know what's best for the organization. You know branding, you've done the work, you know the market; and after all, it's your organization, and it's up to you to set the direction for the future.

Final thoughts on the brand strategy development process

In considering the brand strategy process, patience is perhaps your most important virtue. The discussions and decisions surrounding core brand elements can get messy, and you need to allow your team time to incubate ideas and let concepts gel. A typical brand strategy process might take three months, not including additional research that may be needed up-front. But don't be surprised if it stretches to six months or even a year. Brand strategies are critical to the long-term success of an organization, and they must be given their due. Although the process should have structured time frames, don't push decisions simply to meet artificial deadlines. It's important that there is consensus among the branding team, and if that means an additional month or two to consider key aspects, the process needs to allow for the additional time.

In addition, when the process is complete, you may look at your brand promise and attributes and feel a sense of buyer's remorse. "We just spent six months and how many dollars to come up with a brand attribute of 'caring'? Isn't that obvious?" However, as with many processes of this nature, there is as much value or more in the thinking that is generated during the process as there is in the outcome. Sure, you may end up in a place that you could have predicted from the beginning. But you've confirmed that decision through a well-thought-through process, which should give you and your leadership the confidence to move forward with enthusiasm. It's often interesting to show a sample brand promise to a CEO or other executive at the beginning of the process. Often, the response is "That just seems like blah, blah, blah," or "Couldn't you apply that statement to any hospital?" From the outside, these perceptions of a brand promise may be true. But when your team goes through the hard work of developing your own brand promise, it becomes yours and it has tremendous meaning for those involved in the process. That meaning is what provides a sense of ownership, which allows the brand strategy to take its rightful place as a highly valued organizational strategy. The next challenge, as we'll see in Chapter 8, is to transfer that meaning and sense of ownership to the rest of the organization.

Living the brand

The process of developing a brand strategy can be exhausting and time-consuming. After months of hard work, sometimes contentious dialogue, and deep, right-brained thinking, a brand strategy is crafted and the formal development process comes to a close. At that point, it's understandable if those involved feel a sense of closure, breathe a sigh of relief, and congratulate one another on a job well done. But of course, the job isn't complete. In fact, it's just beginning. If developing a brand strategy is like pregnancy and giving birth, the work of living the brand is like the work of raising that child from infancy to adulthood. And often, it takes just as long.

In this chapter, we'll look at the aspects of launching the brand-building effort and maintaining the work over time. As with the process of developing the brand strategy, there are nearly limitless ways to approach ongoing brand-building work. After all, this is organizational change at its grandest level, and brand-building can extend to all corners of an organization. You should consider the steps and tools in this chapter as a basic outline of how to approach brand-building, and you are encouraged to explore other sources for insight and inspiration. The more you're exposed to different strategies and tactics, the more likely you are to land on the approaches that work best for you and your organization. In the end, there's only one guarantee: The only strategy that absolutely will not work is to do nothing at all.

Brand-building roles

Ask who is responsible for living the brand in an organization, and the answer you'll often hear is "everyone." This is true in the purest sense, as everyone in a provider organization, from the CEO to the physician to the night janitor, impacts the brand. However, it would be clearly ineffective to simply hand out the brand strategy document to all employees and say, "Now start living the brand." Although everyone will have a role to play, three specific jobs must be fulfilled to ensure a successful brand-building effort: brand champion, brand manager, and the brand council.

The brand champion

Finding the brand champion in any healthcare organization is the easy part—it's the CEO, the administrator, or whoever holds the top executive title. For branding to fulfill its potential, it must be championed by the top executive. This ensures that branding will always receive the attention, the urgency, the focus, the priority, and the resources it deserves. But that doesn't mean the brand champion does all the heavy lifting. Given that the responsibility falls to the person in the organization with perhaps more demands on his or her time than any other, the actual workload of the brand champion is lighter than one might expect. But the importance of that work is vital.

The brand champion's primary responsibility is to be the organization's voice of the brand. That is, the brand champion should extol the elements of the brand at every opportunity, both internally and externally. In some cases, that will involve outlining the explicit wording of the brand strategy, such as in an employee training session. In other cases, it will mean reinforcing a key brand attribute, such as tying the announcement of the opening of a new primary care clinic during a groundbreaking ceremony speech to the organization's focus on providing "convenient" care. Because the top administrator oversees all aspects of the organization, he or she has the best opportunity to tie brand in across all services, in more places than anyone else could.

The brand champion also gives authority to the brand, which is another reason this role must be served by the top executive, who has final decision-making power in many situations. Following the brand strategy will require setting priorities and focusing on some areas while putting off others. That requires saying no to a funding request, or a director's desire to add staff, or a physician's demand for some sort of special treatment. Saying no in those situations because of brand priorities often will be ill-received, and the person making the request may try to go higher in the organization to seek approval. If the brand champion is a manager or director, another member of the organization may be able to pull rank and push the request through despite the negative brand implications. With the CEO serving as brand champion, the organization is assured that the top executive understands and values brand

and will take the brand strategy into consideration when tough decisions are made. The brand champion also can provide authority by ensuring that branding efforts are funded, whether for training, communications, or special initiatives that may have little short-term benefit but could go a long way toward building a strong brand.

The brand manager

The title *brand manager* can mean different things in different organizations. In some cases, brand management refers to those responsible within the organization for maintaining corporate identity standards (often disparagingly referred to as the brand police, or worse). For our purposes, we'll define the brand manager as the person who is responsible for ensuring that brand-building strategies are advanced throughout the organization. While receiving support from the CEO as brand champion and a brand council, the brand manager is responsible for the heavy lifting of brand-building. If branding is a function of the organization, the brand manager is the functional leader. The brand manager owns the work of bringing the brand strategy to life, executing the desires and decisions of the brand council, and working with other leaders to build brand throughout the organization.

Typically, the brand manager is a marketing or new business development executive. Sometimes it's the top executive, such as a vice president or chief marketing officer. Other times, it could be a director-level marketing executive, reporting to a higher marketing executive but owning the brand-building work. Depending on the size of the organization, there may be a position dedicated solely to brand management at a director or even vice president level. In some larger systems, there may even be a team of brand managers. Often, however, the responsibility of brand management is shared with marketing or similar responsibilities.

The brand manager role requires a unique set of qualifications. Although the needs will vary by organization, a strong brand manager has:

- A fundamental understanding of brand
- The vision and ability to articulate the brand strategy
- Collaborative/facilitative skills
- Determination and energy
- Effective public speaking skills
- Initiative and drive
- Resilience
- Proficiency in project management
- Experience in launching and building brands

As with finding a branding consultant, hiring a brand manager who is familiar with healthcare but also has experience outside of healthcare is preferred.

The brand council

In many organizations, a brand council is created to oversee ongoing brand-building efforts. The brand council lends advice and direction to the CEO, helping to make tough brand-related decisions and setting the course of action for specific brand-building initiatives. The brand council may be the same team that helped to develop the brand strategy, or a new group may be created. In some smaller organizations, the leadership team itself becomes the brand council by default. In addition to driving brand-building initiatives and supporting decisions related to branding, the brand council members should serve as brand disciples throughout the organization. That is, they should be true believers who, like the CEO, champion the brand in their areas of influence. Thus, the brand council may include top executives, leading physicians, board members with a specific expertise or interest in brand, or others who are in a position of influence within the organization.

Others throughout the organization may also play important roles related to brand. As mentioned before, communications executives responsible for managing corporate identity standards are an example. Often, those in the marketing communications department play an extended role with branding, given the focus on external brand communications and the natural inclination of those in this department to understand and value brand.

Organizations frequently engage outside consultants, branding firms, or creative agencies to serve a brand support role. Most often these partnerships exist in the arena of external brand communications, such as the development of marketing communications materials, the design and maintenance of a Web site, or the creation of advertising campaigns. Some consultants also serve as a proxy brand manager, providing ideas, insights, and honest feedback to the internal brand manager, the brand champion, and/or the brand council in various capacities. Although outside consultants can provide wonderful support, the ownership of building the brand must remain an internal function, for the sake of both continuity and credibility. Just as with raising a child, there are all manners of childcare, therapists, or counselors who can help, but it's up to the parents to carry the load.

The brand launch

Once a brand strategy is developed and key brand roles are filled, it's time for the launch, but not the type of launch you may be thinking of. This isn't a big, splashy advertising campaign or the unveiling of a new slogan. Before any external brand communication, the brand strategy must be introduced internally. In some cases, there may be no reason to even generate external brand-focused communications. For example, perhaps there may be too much to do in the area of living the brand promise before it is ready for public promotion.

Unfortunately, many organizations rush to communicate their brand values, either out of excitement from the new strategy or because a branding campaign was the goal all along, and the brand strategy was seen simply as a necessary step in the campaign development. Always remember that brands are built first and foremost by the experiences your consumers have, not by communicated brand messages. That means you must be delivering the brand experiences you desire, and that means ensuring that everyone in the organization knows what those are.

The internal launch effort can include many components, but the order of events is important to maximize success. For starters, the brand council must be brought up to speed on the brand strategy, its meaning, and how it will be brought to life (assuming this is a different group than those responsible for developing the brand strategy). In addition, any of the brand council members who don't have a complete or consistent understanding of branding must be brought up to speed, as they will be seen as the senior leaders of the branding efforts and must be able to respond to questions and concerns from others. Efforts to educate brand council members can be directed by the brand manager, an outside consultant, or both.

Next, organizational leaders who have yet to have any exposure to the brand strategy need to be introduced to the concept. Often, this can take place in the form of "Branding 101" sessions, where either the brand manager, members of the brand council, or an outside consultant gives executives at the vice president and director levels a crash course in branding, introduces the organization's brand strategy, and outlines the role that branding will play moving forward. Depending on the size of the organization, managers may be included in this step as well, or they may be given a separate introduction, either by their directors or by the brand manager.

At this point, the brand strategy is ready for introduction to the entire organization. This can be handled in a number of ways. The question of whether introduction to the brand strategy is mandatory for all employees is still open. Some experts believe that brand-building involvement should be voluntary, and adding one more, rarely understood initiative to the plate of the frontline worker is too much to ask. Others would say that if you truly want to leverage the value of branding, everyone who can impact the brand must understand what is expected of him or her. You will need to decide based on your culture, leadership style, and experience with launching large, organization-wide initiatives which approach will work best for you.

Some organizations hold large events, such as a series of town-hall-style meetings led by the CEO. In other cases, employees are introduced to the brand strategy in small groups, by department or specific area. No matter how the staff is approached, it's critical that organizational managers have already been introduced to the brand strategy and have been given ample opportunity to ask questions and seek clarification. For many on the staff, whether they are physicians, nurses, or administrative workers, branding will be a completely foreign concept, and many will turn to their managers for further explanation and insight.

Throughout the launch process, a number of tools can be used, whether initially with the brand council or with frontline workers. First, the brand book should be a tool that's available to anyone, though you can decide whether to automatically distribute it to everyone in the organization. At a minimum, copies should be available for those who are interested, either in printed form or for download off your intranet. Also, keep in mind the various diverse audiences you employ. You may need to create a version in a different language depending on your employee mix.

Many organizations also create a distinct section on their Web site, either the external site (that is password-protected) or on their intranet, where the brand strategy elements reside. The benefit of this tool is that the content can be extended as much as necessary or updated whenever needed without additional production costs. For example, a Web-based brand section is an excellent means for updating brand embodiment points, and it can become a repository for organizational stories that help to support the brand. Taken further, a Web site can house training tools, such as orientation videos or "brand exams" that test employee knowledge of organizational brand elements. Review of the brand section of the Web site can be part of a new-employee orientation, or can even be built into continuing education programs.

Other tools include printed pieces that help to remind the staff of the key brand elements. Existing internal communications vehicles, such as an organization-wide newsletter or departmental informational memos, can be leveraged. Although distribution of the brand book may be on an as-requested basis, perhaps all employees are given a one-page overview of the brand strategy, or some other useful reminder, such as a poster, calendar, or wallet card. Of course, any communications piece needs to be considered in concert with other core organizational initiatives. For example, many hospitals and health systems print their mission, values, or service standards on their identification badges, making the addition of brand strategy elements unwieldy or downright confusing.

Ongoing brand embodiment efforts

With a brand strategy in place and communicated throughout the organization, the ongoing work of building the brand can truly begin. There are two primary ways to drive brand embodiment throughout the organization: "push" strategies and "pull" strategies. A mix of both push and pull strategies will help to ensure that you are maximizing your brand-building efforts.

Push strategies

Push strategies, often driven from the top down, involve proactively taking the brand strategy and generating ideas for how the organization might better live its brand, and then pushing those ideas down through the organization to completion. For example, the brand council might spend half a day brainstorming new services that could be introduced to help to better embody the organization's brand attribute of "convenient." Perhaps the organization will create a branded mini clinic to put in local supermarkets or add a drive-through pharmacy, or institute a 30-minute guarantee in the ER. The ideas are flushed out and then those with merit go through the appropriate channels for exploration and development.

The benefit of creating push strategies is that they often allow participants to think outside the normal planning channels, focusing only on how to enhance the brand. This will lead to ideas that otherwise may never have been considered. Push strategies are also beneficial in that they can jumpstart brand-building efforts. Creating a mini clinic, for example, or a 30-minute ER guarantee, will ensure that the organization is continuing to build its brand and will provide evidence that the organization is serious about its direction.

The downside of push strategies is that because they're developed outside the normal organizational planning streams, they are harder to make a reality. First, the initiative must find a home, and not everyone will be happy to be given a new initiative that has been "pushed" down on them from above. Not everyone at a functional level will believe in the value of the initiative, and they might even handicap the project because it competes for financial resources with a manager's own priorities.

One way around this is to engage functional or departmental leaders in developing push strategies to support brand-building at their level. For example, as part of the normal annual or budgeting process, the brand manager can work with a service line leader to brainstorm ways in which the department could further embody the organizational brand. The presence of the brand manager helps to focus the thinking around brand-building, but participating managers have control over which initiatives they support.

Pull strategies

The term *pull strategy* refers to the identification and prioritization of existing ideas or initiatives that best support brand-building efforts, which are then prioritized and "pulled" through the process faster. For example, the director of surgery may create an annual operational plan based on volume goals, physician requests, and key organizational initiatives such as safety or customer service. Then, with the help of the brand manager, or using the tools that help to communicate the brand strategy elements, the director tags those initiatives or requests that best support the brand and gives those priority. Or perhaps the brand manager collects those priority initiatives, along with all the other brand priority initiatives throughout the organization, and takes them to the brand council, where a special "brand-building" budget is applied to the best initiatives, providing the functional leaders with additional funding or support to make the initiatives a reality.

The benefit of pull strategies is that because they emanate from existing planning streams, they are more likely to become a reality. Because they were initiated by a departmental director or manager, there's a sense of ownership, and their value is inherent to these leaders. On the downside, pull strategies require the understanding and valuing of brand-building efforts by directors and managers, which isn't always present. It also requires their ability to recognize potential brand-building priorities, unless the brand manager is available to help. Finally, because pull strategies come from traditional planning processes, they are less likely to represent new thinking, or truly differentiating ideas.

The brand gap analysis

To successfully identify potential push or pull strategies, it's often important to conduct a brand gap analysis at a functional or clinical level. The purpose of a brand gap analysis is to determine the disparity between the desired brand and the experience currently delivered. Although you undoubtedly can find some of this information in the findings report issued in the brand strategy process, that research typically looks at the brand from an organizational perspective, not from a specific functional or clinical perspective.

Take, for example, the desired brand attribute of "convenient," and then consider a heart center. When it comes to delivering convenient heart care, what does this look like? How convenient is the heart care now, compared to what it could be? Depending on the attribute, a brand gap analysis can become fairly complex. For example, what if a brand promise revolved around providing the most advanced care available to the market? When considering cardiology, understanding what "the most advanced care" means is having a vision of that promise related to cardiology, understanding new advances in technology or drug treatments, and knowing which procedures are considered "advanced" and which are considered "experimental."

Conducting a brand gap analysis may require outside help, someone who understands the clinical arena well enough and can look beyond the opinions of a particularly egotistical heart surgeon or the basic information available on consumer Web sites to truly map the brand gap, and the opportunities that exist for building the brand in that specific area. The same thinking could be applied to human resources, information technology, and other functional areas as well.

Managing external brand communications

The bulk of this book is devoted to outlining how to build brands within an organization, and we've made an explicit point of separating brand communications as a subcomponent of branding, but not as branding itself. But now it's time to give some key elements of external communications their due, because in addition to simply carrying a branding message, the communications themselves can help to shape your brand. In other words, perception can help to shape reality.

A Marketer's Guide to Brand Strategy

A great example of the power that communications can have in shaping brand perception is an organization's name. Although developing a brand strategy isn't inherently about changing the company name, the process often leads to just such a result. If you want your brand to be valued in a certain way and your name doesn't support that desired brand, or worse, it contradicts it, a change may be required. For example, if you want to be valued as the first choice for care in a region, but your name features the town in which your hospital is located, it will be harder for those outside that community to value you as their first choice. Or perhaps you want to be valued for the convenience your system offers, yet you have a product-oriented branding hierarchy, which means that each facility carries its own, independent name. In that case, it's hard for consumers to give you credit for multiple locations—one important aspect of convenience—if they can't easily connect all of your locations as part of one offering.

In fact, the power of a unified brand hierarchy (in addition to making brand awareness much easier on the consumer) is its potential to knock down internal walls and silos. Many systems, for example, are composed of facilities that were acquired over the years, and in many cases were allowed to keep their original names. Although there is often equity in a hospital's traditional name within its community, in some cases the different names help to support the mentality of "us versus them." Take a system that has multiple hospitals within the same metropolitan area, where the impact of historical reputations and the small-town, "hometown" mindset are lessened. "We always are successful with our cardiac programs, but City Hospital always gets more credit." Having all facilities under the same name, as members of the same family (as opposed to feeling like in-laws), removes a powerful and emotional barrier to those facilities actually acting as members of the same family. And this helps your organization to deliver a more consistent brand experience, and in all likelihood, a consistently better brand experience.

The issue of naming and brand embodiment also becomes important with issues of cobranding. There are many benefits to cobranding your organization with sponsors, partner physician groups, affiliated organizations, or others. But in addition to often causing confusion among consumers, organizations must be careful in attaching their name to brand experiences they can't control.

Like an organization's name, its corporate identity can shape how the brand is perceived in the market. If you desire to be valued as a modern, progressive organization, but your logo hasn't changed since 1974 and your corporate colors are outdated, it will be difficult for the market to perceive you as modern or progressive, even if you have a new facility or the latest technology. The same goes with your advertising, Web site, marketing communications materials, and more. Many of these elements may need to change, in both content and style, to accurately reflect your desired brand.

Final thoughts on living the brand

In the end, moving your organization to truly live its desired brand is classic change management. A whole industry is dedicated just to this concept, with hundreds of books and thousands of authors, experts, and consultants in change management. One of the best is John Kotter from Harvard Business School, one of the most recognized experts on leadership and change. Two of his books, *Leading Change* and *The Heart of Change,* are must reads for anyone engaging in a brand-building effort. But a number of standard principles to approaching change management are helpful to remember as you work to build your organization's brand.

Communication is critical

To put it bluntly, you cannot communicate enough when it comes to internal brand-building. On the topic of change management, Kotter estimates that most organizations undercommunicate change by "a factor of ten." Another famed expert on the subject insists that for a message to sink in, it must be communicated "seven times in seven different ways." Often, leaders in an organization fall into a trap of assuming that because they've been talking about brand for a year, everyone else must have spent an equal amount of time considering the concept. Or they get tired of delivering the same message over and over. But the old saying in communications rings true: Just when you're getting sick of the message you're delivering, your audience is just beginning to get it. Branding can be reinforced through traditional internal communications, or vehicles dedicated solely to promoting the brand can be developed. Information can include updated brand measurements, individual stories or other brand embodiment points, and examples of successes achieved in brand-building.

What gets measured gets done

The management principle of "what gets measured gets done" applies to brand-building as well as any initiative or strategy. In the next chapter, we'll look at ways to measure the effectiveness of brand-building efforts. But as I've outlined in this chapter, for branding to maximize its value, it takes an organization-wide effort, which means that supporting the brand must be important to each individual. You can preach the value of brand to employees, but if their performance isn't measured against brand-related goals, it's unlikely they will strive to support the brand. Work with your human resources leader to develop a means for building the brand strategy into job descriptions and performance measurement objectives so that salary increases, advancement, and other rewards are tied to building the brand.

Clear the decks

Large strategic initiatives such as brand-building require time and resources. However, these new demands can't be additive. If you expect employees to simply add brand-building efforts to their already full plates, you'll be in for disappointment. The same goes for budgets. If an initiative calls for adding mini clinics, the money has to come from somewhere. For brand-building to be successful, priorities have to be set and tough decisions have to be made. Leadership must "clear the decks" of lower priorities to allow for the pursuit and implementation of branding initiatives and efforts. Identifying and categorizing elements as lower priorities is never easy. Without making the hard choices, however, branding will, at best, provide only incremental value.

References

Kotter, John P. *Leading Change* (Harvard Business School Press: 1996), p. 9.

Kaplan, Robert S., and David P. Norton. *Alignment: Using the Balance Scorecard to Create Corporate Synergies* (Harvard Business School Press: 2006), p. 87.

Challenges to brand-building

As you begin the journey to make your brand strategy a reality, you'll face any number of challenges along the way. Five in particular tend to cause the most problems for those building brands in healthcare, from lack of understanding and buy-in to new-program burnout.

A fundamental lack of understanding of brand

We've hit this point throughout the book, but it bears repeating yet again. The vast majority of your organization will have little or no understanding of brand, which poses a huge challenge to brand-building success. It starts with your leadership—a brand strategy is simply wishful thinking if your CEO or administrator isn't on board. Though you shouldn't expect other organizational leaders to necessarily understand branding—from the COO to the CFO to the CIO—the more you have to work to bring them up to speed, the longer and more painful it will be to make your brand strategy effective.

Once you enter the organization at large, all bets are off. Branding will be completely foreign to most, and those that do know of branding will most likely have the wrong idea of it. Although it's hard to educate someone who has no background in a particular concept, it's even harder to re-educate someone who has a misunderstanding of that concept.

As you move through your brand-building efforts, keep an eye out for the misconceptions and myths outlined in Chapters 4 and 5. Prepare talking points that help to clarify each, and generate a bibliography of resources that others can access for more information on branding. As new employees enter the organization, you'll find the education process to be a constant challenge.

Branding often loses out to hard capital expenditures

One result of the misunderstanding of branding in healthcare is how it's treated financially. A senior marketing executive at a midsize health system once relayed his struggles in funding his branding and service-related initiatives. Because the cost of these various initiatives—which included an identity redesign, a Customer Relationship Management initiative, and other projects—was significant, the budgeting process called for them to be reviewed by the organization's "capital committee." The capital committee was charged with reviewing all budget requests for the coming fiscal year above a certain expense level. All such requests were put on a list, and the committee debated the items and prioritized them by need. A line was drawn on the list representing the cut-off point: All requests above the line were approved and anything below was declined. At the end of this process, all of the marketing executive's initiatives were below the line. In fact, not a single request above the line related to branding, the patient experience, service, or research. The items that were approved were hard capital costs, such as equipment, facility improvements, and more.

It's not difficult to imagine scenes such as this playing out in hospitals and health systems across the country. Part of the reason soft costs such as branding and experience innovation are still not valued is that businesses as a whole are slow to value these soft assets. *Business Week*'s chief economist, Michael Mandel, floats the premise that the U.S. economy is stronger than most experts believe because the measurements used to gauge the economy are rooted in outdated, manufacturing-oriented thinking. Mandel posits that the government's decades-old system of number collection and crunching captures investments in equipment, buildings, and software, but for the most part misses the growing portion of U.S. gross domestic product (GDP) that is generating the cool, game-changing ideas.

In his argument, Mandel estimates that annually, more than $1 trillion in investments in innovation, product design, brand-building, employee training, or research is not counted in estimates of the GDP. This would represent nearly 8% of the 2006 GDP. Why is the economy measured in such a way that would miss these elements? Mandel gives two key reasons for this misguided thinking. First, the basis for measuring today's economy was created in the 1930s and 1940s, in large part as a reaction to the Great Depression and World War II. Leaders of the Industrial Age wanted to know how the United States was progressing through these events, and measurements were created that counted machines and buildings, but not education or branding. Despite the changes in our economy to a knowledge-based industry, nothing has really changed.

Second, as we'll discuss in the next chapter, soft investments are notoriously hard to measure. How does one capture the true value of brand-building, or training, or innovation research, when the tangible benefits are so difficult to identify? Of course, just because they're hard to quantify doesn't mean these investments don't have value, but it makes it difficult to include them in measuring the economy.

All of this brings us back to our example of the frustrated marketing executive who found all of his projects below the cut-off line. Think of the reasons just explained for this old-school measurement of our economy and then apply them to the brand manager's job in healthcare of proving the value of branding. The organization's method for measuring value is based on hard investments, not soft costs. It's difficult, if not impossible, to measure the ROI of something such as a new corporate identity. Your leaders are often hard-wired to value CT scanners and new hospital wings, not something that's soft and squishy like branding.

The solution to this dilemma is twofold. First, you must embark on the long path of re-educating your leadership in this area. Second, you must be patient and give your leaders time to rethink the old ways and begin to value branding for what it can truly bring to the organization.

A Marketer's Guide to Brand Strategy

The ADP syndrome

A friend of mine once told the story of his experience working with a health system to develop and communicate an organizational vision. During an open forum with directors and managers, he noticed one middle-aged man sitting with his arms crossed, clearly not buying into the message being delivered. After the session, the consultant asked the man what he was thinking about:

"ADP," the man said.

"What is ADP?" asked the consultant.

"ADP: another damn program," the man said. "I've outlasted other efforts like this, and I'll outlast this one too."

Here was an employee who was so burned out by corporate initiatives that he refused to even consider engaging with a new one.

Unfortunately, odds are that a segment of your internal audience suffers from ADP syndrome. Corporations have great intentions in developing initiatives, programs, and organizational philosophies, and we can all name the most recent and most common: mission, vision, strategic planning, Six Sigma, Lean Manufacturing, Lean Six, service standards, innovation, quality, safety. The list goes on and on, and now we're adding branding to the mix. With the quantity of initiatives and the way they are often mishandled, it's no wonder employees grow numb to the idea of change.

Of course, that doesn't mean your organization should stop trying to improve or to roll out new initiatives. But it does highlight the challenge of adding brand-building to the plate of already overwhelmed employees. They must know that the brand strategy is for real, why it's important, and that leadership supports it. They need to understand that their performance will be measured against brand values, and that branding will have a positive impact on what they care about most—their patients. Discipline, consistency, constant communication, continual feedback, and the celebration of successes all help employees to overcome ADP syndrome and begin to engage in brand-building.

What have you done for me lately?

Today, corporate cultures are often focused on immediate results, which often come at the expense of tomorrow's success. We all know the drill. Maybe it's cutting marketing expenses this quarter to make the numbers, which will have a negative impact on volumes the next quarter. Or perhaps new hires are postponed to lower expenses, leading to a drop in customer service levels. Whatever the strategy, sacrificing tomorrow's potential for today's gain can become a vicious cycle of always trying to play catch-up. The situation is worse for publicly held companies, which must meet the quarterly projections of industry analysts or see their stock prices take a hit.

Usually, the CEO or administrator feels the most pressure to improve today's situation, and understandably so. But more and more, marketing leaders also are feeling the pressure. In fact, research shows that of all the senior positions in a corporation, the chief marketing officer has the shortest shelf live, with an average of only 26 months on the job. In healthcare, more and more is expected from these executives, and the misunderstanding of branding and marketing in general that is pervasive in healthcare only compounds the issue. This pressure to show results now can stop brand-building in its tracks. Branding is a long-term investment in the future success of an organization. As we've discussed, it can take years for true brand-building efforts to take hold. Because it's hard to show ROI on many branding initiatives, it makes it easier for executives to reject them.

When it comes to branding, this issue results from a combination of issue one, a lack of understanding, and issue three, a lack of seeing branding as a worthy investment. Addressing those issues will go a long way toward helping your organization accept the long-term investment that is branding.

Leadership turnover

Maybe the number-one reason brand strategies fail is lack of consistent leadership. As we just read, the position with the most turnover at the executive level is the CMO. Right behind that position is the CEO, whose average turnover is 44 months. These, of course, are the two most important positions in the organization when it comes to developing and leading a brand strategy. The loss of either one of these executives can doom brand-building efforts. Often, new hires want to make a fresh start or make their own mark on the organization, which drives them to change top strategies such as branding. Or perhaps they don't understand or value branding, or they feel it should be a lower priority for the organization.

What makes this challenge so daunting is that there is little you can do to prevent leadership turnover. Leaders change for all sorts of reasons, but in the end, it's the rare organization that is able to keep its two top branding leaders together for five or 10 years. Nevertheless, the value of branding is too great for organizations to abandon the strategy because of this challenge. The more inclusive the brand strategy development process, the more comprehensive the brand strategy launch, and the more embedded the brand-building efforts, the greater the likelihood that brand-building can continue should the CEO or top marketing executive move on.

References

Mandel, Michael. "Why the Economy Is a Lot Stronger Than You Think." *BusinessWeek*, February 13, 2006.

David Kiley and Burt Helm. "The Short Life of the Chief Marketing Officer." *BusinessWeek*, December 10, 2007.

David Kiley and Burt Helm. "The Short Life of the Chief Marketing Officer." *BusinessWeek*, December 10, 2007.

Measuring your progress

As I demonstrated in Chapter 1, building a strong brand leads to greater success for organizations over time. The trick, of course, is to demonstrate the impact of branding efforts on an individual organization—your organization. Measuring the effectiveness of your brand strategy is a significant challenge for a number of reasons:

- Brands take time to build. If you've created a brand strategy and have begun the hard work of moving your organization toward living that desired brand, how long must you wait to see results? Some changes may show up in a matter of weeks or months, and these successes should be celebrated to demonstrate the ongoing power of branding. But achieving your desired brand strategy—having your market over-whelmingly value you based on the promise and attributes you desire—can take years. It can be extraordinarily difficult to measure something as complicated as branding over that period of time. People change, measurement methods change, strategies and tactics change. Sometimes even key aspects of the brand strategy may change. All of which make it difficult to show results over time.

- It's hard to isolate the impact of branding. Along with potentially taking years to see a significant impact, branding affects all aspects of an organization. Both of these realities make it extremely difficult to isolate brand-building efforts from other causes shaping an outcome. Was the five-year period of positive income due to branding efforts, a new COO, or a robust U.S. economy? No doubt, all three causes, and many others, played a role. But how do leaders carve out the impact of branding to know whether they're taking the right steps, or whether the impact of their strategies is having any effect?

- Most organizations lack a stock price to use as a guide. Research has proven that companies with strong brands realize a greater stock valuation, providing a consistent metric for measuring brands. A few healthcare providers are public companies, and therefore can use stock price as a core measurement for their brand. But the vast majority of hospitals and health systems are not public, and so have no stock price to gauge.

The brand dashboard

Although these challenges are real enough, that doesn't excuse a brand manager from developing methods to measure the effectiveness of branding efforts. It's absolutely crucial to the sustainability of a brand strategy to have a legitimate, ongoing means of measuring success. One solution is to create a brand dashboard, or a set of standardized measurements, to provide a benchmark for the brand. One value of a dashboard approach is that the metrics are updated regularly and are easily disseminated throughout the organization. A report can be quickly created showing the latest dashboard results for a board meeting, or an update to the brand council. Some organizations may create a Web-based dashboard that can provide a real-time snapshot of the value of the brand.

Not only does a brand dashboard provide easy access to up-to-date measurements of the organizational brand, but it will also allow a brand manager to track how the brand fluctuates given certain occurrences over time. For instance, how does the brand dashboard look after the organization's annual fundraising gala? Do metrics improve, stay static, or trend negative? After a few years of tracking this data, a brand manager may be able to predict the impact of such an event on the organizational brand. The same method can be used to help measure the impact on brand of advertising campaigns, community educational events, positive or negative stories in the press, the distribution of a community newsletter, the completion of a service initiative, and so on.

A brand dashboard consists of any number of measurable elements, broken down into simple outputs. For example, the results of the annual community perception survey might be boiled down to the response on one question, such as "How willing are you to recommend XYZ Hospital to family and friends?" The brand dashboard might show the percentage of people who responded with the top response of "very willing," or it might show a ratio of top responses versus bottom responses (80/6 equals 80% answered "very willing" and 6% answered "not willing at all"). In addition to showing the actual metric, some dashboards will use color-coding to reflect the comparison of actual data to the organization's goals and objectives. If the organization had set a goal of 90% for those whose response was "very willing," the dashboard would show the actual metric of 80% in red. Had the response been 92%, the metric would have been shown in green. Using simple color-coding helps to easily communicate the metrics, and it adds a level of emotion to the dashboard. A dashboard report that comes back all red will certainly cry out for attention.

Of course, setting measurable objectives can be a challenge. What should be the expected number of respondents answering "very willing to recommend" on a survey? How should branding efforts impact that? For many metrics, benchmarks exist and can be found in industry literature or in resources provided by industry associations. Although it's important to strive to set measurable objectives whenever possible (remember, what gets measured gets done), another approach is to simply measure positive and negative trends. In this case, a "green" result simply means the metric is positive compared to the last measurement, whereas a "red" result indicates a negative outcome.

Which measurements should you include in your brand dashboard? There are potentially dozens of ways to measure the impact of your brand-building efforts. There are four ways to categorize the resources for gathering results.

Audience behavior measurements

Tracking audience behaviors is perhaps the most important measuring stick for your brand. In the end, you care far less about what your key constituencies say than about what they do. After all, the ultimate purpose of your branding efforts is to induce loyal usage of your services from your key audiences. Audience behavior measurements can include:

- Inpatient volumes or admissions
- Outpatient visits/physician office visits
- Surgical cases
- Visits to the ED
- Physician referrals
- Market share data
- Attendance at screenings or classes
- Donation levels
- Call center activity
- Web site visits
- Requests for information
- Ethnographic studies (the science of observing behavior)

Audience attitudes

A close second to audience behaviors in measuring the impact of branding is audience attitudes. How do your audiences feel about your organization? How do they value it? These metrics help you to gauge how the market's perception of your organization is aligning with your desired brand values. Attitudes are second to behaviors because expressed opinions don't always correlate to expected behavior. Just because someone says he or she would refer you to a friend doesn't mean he or she ever has, or ever will. Still, measuring audience attitudes can help to paint a complete picture when it comes to measuring your branding efforts. Examples of measurements of audience attitudes include:

- Community surveys measuring awareness, preference, and perception
- Patient satisfaction surveys
- Physician surveys
- E-mail or online surveys
- Advertising recognition/recall research
- "How did you hear of us?" surveys of patients and consumers (such as those registering for a class)
- Focus groups
- One-on-one interviews, including metaphor-based interviews
- Patient stories
- Staff anecdotes
- Feedback from comment cards or suggestion boxes

Third-party opinions

Assessing how third parties perceive your organization is becoming an increasingly vital measurement of brand value for healthcare providers. With the rise of consumer-driven healthcare, consumers are being asked to spend more of their own money to receive care. As with other expenditures, they will begin to consider the entire spectrum of value, from access and expertise to service, convenience, and price. As they consider the multitude of factors that go into making a healthcare decision, consumers are turning to sources other than providers for help.

The mass of resources available to consumers on healthcare is mind-boggling. For healthcare providers, it's important to begin to monitor these resources to see how your brand is reflected. In some cases, such as "top hospital" awards, specific actions on your part can directly impact the outcome. In others, such as with patient advocates, the entirety of your brand will come into play. Third-party opinions that reflect your brand include:

- Health information resources, such as WebMD
- Health ratings services, such as HealthGrades
- Health industry awards/rankings, such as Thomson's "Top 100 Hospitals," or J.D. Power rankings, or *U.S. News & World Report*'s annual top hospitals list
- Health research companies, such as the National Research Corporation
- Accreditation resources, such as The Joint Commission
- Provider comparison Web sites, often hosted by payers, governmental groups such as CCS, or state hospital associations
- Patient story Web sites
- Social networks, such as MySpace and Facebook
- Bloggers
- Traditional print and broadcast media
- Employers
- Health and wellness corporations (that manage programs for employers)

- Patient advocates
- Bond rating companies

Financial metrics

As we've seen, brand-building can have a direct impact on an organization's bottom line. For those few public healthcare providers, stock valuation provides a proven measure for the value of brand. For the rest, there are a number of potential financial metrics to gauge. The challenge with financial metrics is to determine how much of an impact brand-building efforts actually have on financial results. For example, can branding efforts be tied to an improved contribution margin, and if so, how?

Although it may be difficult to tie a branding effort or initiative directly to a financial outcome, these measurements provide the ultimate thermometer for the health of a company. As such, they reflect the overall health of the brand. Financial outcomes can be compared to organization objectives, past performance, or industry benchmarks. Here are some common financial measurements that could be included in the brand dashboard:

- Revenue
- Operating or net income
- Contribution margin
- Income margins
- Debt to asset ratios
- Accounts receivable turnover

- Cash flow/cash on hand
- Balance sheet equity
- Current ratio
- Community benefit statistics

Final thoughts on measuring brand effectiveness

You should consider many variables when measuring brand effectiveness. What should be measured? How is effectiveness or success defined? How often are metrics updated? Who has access to the information? How are variables and anomalies accounted for? It can seem overwhelming at first to find answers to all of these questions. One option is to turn to an outside consultant, who can help you create your brand dashboard. A number of firms also offer proprietary products and systems for measuring brand effectiveness. Or your own research and planning department might be up to the task of creating the brand dashboard. If necessary, start small, looking at just a handful of metrics. Then slowly build your expertise and add more measurements over time. However it is structured, your brand dashboard will be an important tool in demonstrating the value of your brand throughout the organization.

Case studies in healthcare brand strategy

A final thought on brand strategy

Brand-building is perhaps one of the most challenging endeavors a marketing leader can undertake. The work is hard, the risks can be high, and the frustrations can be intense. The journey is flush with pitfalls, and setbacks abound. But the rewards are tremendous, to you as a marketing leader, to your organization's leader, to the organization as a whole, and of course, to the patients you serve. Successful brand-building will help your organization differentiate itself in an increasingly crowded marketplace, allowing you to achieve your vision of success in the future. By definition, it will lead to a better organization and a better experience for those you serve.

In the following three sections, you will find the stories of three healthcare providers who have taken the journey to build better brands. They have valiantly agreed to share their stories to benefit others in similar situations. You won't have access to their complete brand strategies—after all, these are highly proprietary values that are best kept close to the vest. But you will get a peek at some of their brand strategy components. More important, you'll learn about the processes they've followed and the tactics they've tried. You'll hear of successes and setbacks. You'll find common themes, as well as unique situations. Most likely, you will learn as much from their stories as you will from the rest of the book.

As you set off on your difficult journey of brand-building, I leave you with two quotes. The first is a common phrase with unknown origins: "Nothing worthwhile ever comes easy." The second comes from one of the wisest teachers in my life, Yoda, who said: "Do or do not. There is no try."

Case study: Northwest Community Hospital

The drive to build a brand strategy at Northwest Community Hospital (NCH) began with the help of a few key influencers from outside the healthcare industry—its board members. President and CEO Bruce Crowther says that he began to take notice of how a few of his organization's board members would talk passionately about the brands of their own companies.

"I've been in healthcare over 31 years, and my experience has been that not too many hospitals talk about their brand, and really still don't today," says Crowther. "But these board members brought a different perspective. For example, one of our board members went on to Motorola, where brand-building is a passion."

Founded in 1959 and serving the northwest suburbs of Chicago, NCH offers a range of healthcare services through a number of facilities, the largest of which is Northwest Community Hospital, a 488-bed facility located in Arlington Heights, IL. Crowther realized that in a crowded market such as NCH's, branding could provide a way to differentiate his organization. He also recognized consumerism as a growing trend that would force health systems to move beyond the basics of care delivery to provide more demonstrable and differentiated value. From the beginning of the process, it was clear that a brand strategy could have a tremendous impact.

"Early on, we did some community focus groups to test our reputation," remembers Crowther. "We had so many things we were proud of internally, but the market didn't really recognize them. Instead, they said we had the cleanest halls. That's obviously not how you want to be known as a hospital. We knew we could be more proactive in guiding our brand."

Although Crowther is a long-tenured healthcare executive, his somewhat unique background helped him to understand the value of branding. Rather than follow the typical educational path of receiving a degree in health administration, he earned an MBA, which gave him more experience with marketing and branding. He knew that many companies outside of healthcare had successfully employed branding to differentiate themselves, but he wondered whether it was possible to truly differentiate one hospital from another.

"Most hospitals are out there creating white noise—'our machine is better than yours is'," he says. "It's expected that everyone will be a player in quality, safety, and technology. Those are really fundamentally assumed, the price of admission. But is anyone creating great experiences? Instinctively, we thought we could provide better experiences than our competition. The question was can we differentiate ourselves through this? Can we really deliver on it?"

Although Crowther's recognition of the value of branding was instrumental in making the strategy a top priority, building the brand strategy began in earnest when Angela Stefaniu, who currently serves as the vice president of marketing and business development, took on the assignment. Crowther stressed how important it was to have someone who both understood branding and had a passion for it. Although he had pushed the idea of branding before asking Stefaniu to take on the responsibility, it didn't get off the ground until someone with those traits was behind it.

Stefaniu's first move in developing the brand strategy was to find help from outside the organization, as she knew it would be critically important to conduct an objective and comprehensive evaluation of the organization's existing and desired brand position. She conducted a search for a brand consultant, interviewing 12 firms from across the country. The intent was to explicitly avoid a "typical advertising agency," many of which, in Stefaniu's experience, had too much of a bias toward defining an organization's brand strategy primarily through advertising or communications. Eventually, she hired MasterPlan, a consulting firm based in Chicago that had worked with companies such as Harley-Davidson, American Express, and the Home Depot. Stefaniu said it was important to her to find a partner with experience outside of healthcare, who would be able to approach the process from outside the typical hospital perspective.

Building on the research already gathered by NCH, MasterPlan took a deeper dive using metaphor-based interviews with physicians, nurses, and staff. Stefaniu said it was fascinating to see physicians who were asked to sit in a room for an hour, eyes closed, visualizing their work experiences. The results of the discovery process were used as a foundation for a two-day off-site meeting on branding that included approximately 25 key organizational leaders, among them top executives and directors. The group focused on strengths and visioning, using a number of team activities, and together they developed a set of brand drivers. For example, in the research, physicians had bemoaned the loss of connectivity to their colleagues and patients, thanks to movements toward more managed care, greater automation, and more. As a result, "collegiality" emerged as a brand driver for physicians.

For Stefaniu, this initial two-day retreat already was somewhat of a risk. "We knew where we needed to go, but we didn't have a plan from A to Z on how to get there," she says. "We weren't sure how the leaders in our organization would respond to the idea of creating a brand strategy and whether they would embrace the concept. But the results were overwhelmingly positive."

Following the formation of the core brand elements, Stefaniu and her consultants developed a "brand book," a document that outlined seven phases of their branding process, the brand strategy, and the rationale behind the work. Although the piece showed the significance of and set the direction of the brand work, Stefaniu said she learned quickly that it wasn't the only resource the organization would need.

Because a brand strategy can be difficult to comprehend in concrete terms, Stefaniu wanted to create a simple tool that would describe the essence of the brand strategy in a nutshell. She developed a one-page brand strategy outline, which focused on the organization's master brand strategy as well as its sub-branding strategies. This document was used in a half-day brand orientation session with the organization's 70-plus operations directors that took place six months after the initial leadership retreat.

Eventually, an abbreviated version of the brand orientation session was offered to all 4,000 employees in the organization. The session was led by the MasterPlan consultant, as well as another consultant who gained most of his experience working with Disney. The consultant with the Disney background helped employees understand how to put the patient first, using the metaphor of "on-stage" and "off-stage." Stefaniu noted that given the typical healthcare culture, this can be a difficult concept for employees, as their jobs often don't allow them the time or space for "off-stage" interactions. This challenge also extends to more than 800 NCH volunteers who serve in many capacities, and likewise need to understand the organization's brand promise. With branding, she says, it's all about putting the patient first. To help bridge the gap, the team focused on using the concept of "experience," an idea to which everyone seemed better able to relate.

To help aid ongoing learning about the brand throughout the organization, Stefaniu's team created the "NCH Experience Center" which resides on the organization's intranet site. Although still in its initial stages of development, the NCH Experience Center lays out core elements of the brand strategy, such as customer service standards, environmental standards, and communications standards.

"For the marketing department, this tool has been like our version of an electronic medical record," says Stefaniu. "The standards are clearly spelled out along with helpful tools to assist our employees and even business partners in delivering a consistent experience for our customers. It's been extraordinarily useful in communicating the actionable elements of the brand strategy to employees."

Stefaniu credits the emphasis on training as a key to helping to move the brand efforts forward in the organization. Another helpful tool was a visual model her team developed, called the "Brand Realization" model (see Figure CS.1). This one-page visual model shows the many ways in which branding is woven throughout the organization, helping to make the impact of branding more tangible to the staff. She notes that one vice president keeps the diagram under the glass on her desk for easy reference.

FIGURE CS.1 **Brand Realization**

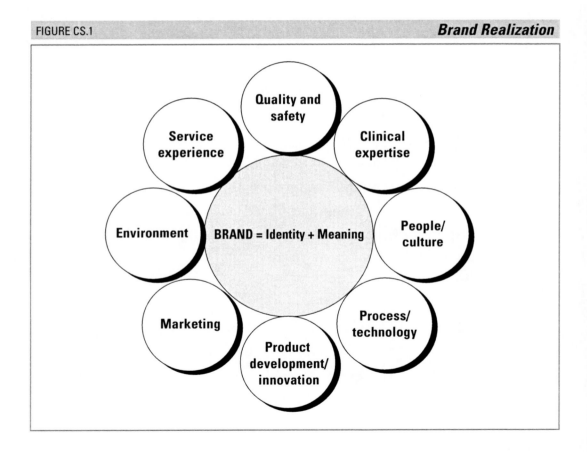

Although these efforts proved valuable to NCH, others didn't fare as well. One example was the creation of a Brand Council, which included 20 people from key operational areas of the organization. Stefaniu says it was hard to engage this group with all the competing priorities they faced. She said the experience taught her that instead of bringing this group together to instill brand in a highly structured way throughout the organization, it was better to empower managers and staff to weave the brand into everyday actions and decisions, using tools such as the Brand Realization model.

Another learning point was the use of storytelling to help demonstrate how the staff could bring the brand strategy to life. Although the idea of story-telling was critical in that regard, says Stefaniu, her team tried to institutionalize the idea through the development and distribution of storytelling kits. The intention was to help educate directors, managers, and team leaders on how best to leverage storytelling, and the goal was to generate stories around a different theme each quarter. After initial success based on feedback from the training sessions and the first wave of storytelling topics, Stefaniu saw the story submissions begin to drop off, and she realized the effort was too much to ask from an organization in the midst of adopting an electronic clinical documentation system and designing an entirely new hospital addition.

"I knew after the second quarter of this program that it would be best to allow the storytelling process to take hold more organically," she says.

One of Stefaniu's team members suggested and designed a storytelling page on the NCH Web site that encourages the exchange of stories from not only employees and volunteers, but also patients and family members.

Whether through storytelling, the use of the Brand Realization model, or via other methods, both Stefaniu and Crowther emphasize the critical role that communication plays in building a brand. As the organization's top leader, Crowther sees one of his most important jobs as constantly reinforcing the brand strategy as a priority. When done right, he says, this can be exhausting.

"As a leader, I'm always thinking about the next new thing, but with change of this scale you have to be consistent with your message over a long period of time," he says. "Essentially, I'm saying the same things over and over, but I can't let that go, I can't get tired of the message. Because even if I'm saying the same thing to a group of employees that I did six months ago, it may be the 100th time I've said it, but it might be only the second time they've heard it."

Not only does Crowther believe that you can't articulate brand values enough, he also says it's vital to consider how these are promoted. At NCH, the brand promise is placed at an equal level to the organization's mission, vision, and values. It is embedded next to them in the organization's strategic plan, and it will soon be incorporated in a financial planning tool for capital requests. The brand strategy is addressed at board retreats and is discussed at the same high level as mission, vision, and strategic planning.

A Marketer's Guide to Brand Strategy

"When discussing brand, it's important that everyone in the organization feels that it is as important as principles like mission or vision," says Crowther. "The brand promise needs to complement these other principles, but they each serve a unique role. It can be challenging for board members or physicians who focus so much on clinical quality or safety to consider brand at the same level. While it's critically important to deliver quality and safety, it's difficult to differentiate your organization with those concepts. When brand is put into context with these other principles we value, then the board members and physicians seem to really embrace it."

In considering how to move a branding effort through an organization, Crowther emphasizes the importance of ensuring that everyone has the same basic understanding of branding and its value. In healthcare, he notes, there is so much misunderstanding of what brand means, but it is still easy to assume that everyone is pointed in the same direction. He gives the example of being halfway through a meeting in the brand strategy process, only to find that a senior leader was taking a totally different perspective, and the group needed to back up and reset the foundation. He says it was helpful to generate an "organizational" definition of brand, which allows individuals to bring different histories and perspectives to the table, but also allows the group to move forward on a common path without anyone thinking someone is wrong. However, he says, it helps to have a culture where employees are given the freedom to interpret the brand values and make them their own. Employees need license to explore ways to serve patients in their own way, to personalize the brand.

Crowther also points out that when discussing a topic as broad as branding, different people would apply different levels of thinking, which could derail the process. For example, he might be discussing high-level strategic concepts, and someone else might enter the conversation at a different level, talking about something such as a logo patch on a uniform. All the levels of thinking are important, he stresses, but keeping everyone at the same level at the same time can be a trick.

Following the extensive internal communications and training process, Stefaniu and her team turned to external communications. The organization took the opportunity to redesign its corporate identity, updating the visual identity system and logo. Although this work helped to emphasize the branding changes, to both external and internal audiences, the identity change did have its drawbacks. As is often the case in identity change, many people had an emotional attachment to the existing look, and Crowther felt that too much hand-wringing was related to the new logo. The initial phase of the external campaign also featured advertising that emphasized the core values of focus for NCH, but as with other advertising efforts, the key for Stefaniu was to walk the walk.

"It's important to our consumers that what they experience when in our care is consistent with what we are promising, that it's real" she says.

The results so far

Measuring the results of their branding efforts has been a challenge, says Crowther. He attributes this in large part to the difficulty in measuring the impact of an improved experience. The organization is currently working to adopt a brand measurement system developed by an instructor from the Northwestern University School of Business, who has developed a proprietary system for measuring brand return on investment. In the meantime, Crowther and Stefaniu point to new ideas that have emerged from the process itself.

In one example, the organization now offers a customized program for mammograms. "Results by Request" enables women to ask for the type of screening appointment they prefer: A 60-minute visit allows a woman to know the results of her exam before she leaves. For women who are comfortable receiving their exam results by mail, a 30-minute appointment option is available. This is one example of providing customers with choice, convenience, and control as it relates to their desired healthcare experience. They've also initiated a significant long-range planning effort to re-conceive the environmental experience, working with a nonprofit group, Project for Public Space, to consider innovative ways to build a connection with their community.

Finally, discussions regarding brand, experience, and consumerism helped to raise the issue of pricing and brought the idea of transparency to the forefront. As a result, NCH became the first in its market to post quality and satisfaction data on its Web site, which led to a positive front-page story in the *Chicago Tribune*. As a result, consumers are requesting more information, looking not just for hospital-wide or service-wide data, but also specific quality data by type of surgery, or even by individual doctor.

"I'm sure eventually we would have come around to transparency, but the brand work made this a much higher priority," says Crowther. "With a brand strategy, so much becomes clear, paths are easier to take, decisions are easier to make. We always talked about the patient experience, but now we're seeing real movement, and that's wholly attributable to our brand-building efforts."

Case study: Borgess Health

Borgess Health is the exception that proves an important brand strategy rule regarding the involvement of the organizational leader in the development process. In summer 2004, Tom Comes, director of marketing and public relations at the Kalamazoo, MI–based health system, began the process of developing a brand strategy. One month after the process began, the organization's CEO left and a number of other C-level positions turned over. Comes and his team were left with a quandary: Wait until new leadership was in place, which might not be for six months, losing the momentum they had generated, or plow forward without a CEO, against conventional wisdom, and pray that the new leader would embrace their direction. As a team, they took a deep breath and decided to move forward.

"End to end, it was a nine-month process, and in the spring of 2005, right when we were wrapping up, a new CEO came on board," says Comes. "I was really sweating bullets. What if he had a completely different take on branding? What if he didn't like the work or the direction we'd chosen? It really gave me the heebie-jeebies."

Fortunately for Comes and his team, the new CEO did like their work. He trusted that the team knew Borgess and its market far better than he did, and that they would know best when it came to the idea of the organization's brand. Although there may be some divine providence in having a new leader come on board with such an open mind, Comes and his team's approach to the brand process had a lot to do with why it had a happy ending. For starters, Comes knew when he started the process that he wasn't looking at creating radically new brand values. Instead, he was considering what he calls a "re-articulation" of the brand.

"Borgess has been around for nearly 120 years, and our brand has evolved over that time through the delivery on our mission and vision," he says. "Our intent wasn't to dramatically change the brand, but rather to measure it in a comprehensive way and then see how we might need to adjust it moving forward. That's why when we presented the brand strategy to the new CEO, it wasn't a shocking departure from what one might expect, which made it easier to embrace."

Comes had been associated with the organization in the 1980s and had participated in initial efforts to tackle brand then. When he returned 20 years later and began to revisit branding, his first step was to hire a strategic partner to manage the brand strategy process. Like Angela Stefaniu at Northwest Community Health, he specifically avoided pure advertising agencies, not wanting any "strings attached" in the form of business opportunities that might result from the brand strategy work. Ultimately, he selected The Strategy Group, based in Norfolk, VA.

The brand strategy process team consisted of Comes, the interim CEO, and four other operational leaders, who met in all-day sessions on a monthly basis. Comes compared the process to moving through a funnel, with discussion of a wide array of issues and possibilities in the beginning that, over time, became more focused. In February 2005, the group had generated the core foundational elements of the brand strategy. From there, the group reviewed a number of brand promise options, finally landing on the one in use today. The process of internally introducing the brand strategy began in June of that year, consisting primarily of small group meetings and one-on-one sessions with employees. External communications reflecting the new brand strategy didn't begin until January of the following year.

Although the process resulted in a brand strategy that the new CEO approved and that met with initial acceptance within the organization, Comes says he might make a few changes if he could do things over again. For one, the brand strategy team did not include a physician. That wasn't an intentional omission— at the time the CMO was one of the executives who'd left, so there were no obvious senior physicians to involve. The concern in adding a physician from one of the system's service areas was that he or she might be too focused in his or her particular field, such as cardiology or neurology. Having a physician's participation on the development team might have led to a smoother rollout, says Comes, but in the end the brand launch was fairly well received. He credits that to revealing the brand strategy to internal staff members and physicians in a way that asked for feedback and input.

"We walked internal staff and physicians through the process, and we didn't present the brand strategy as set in stone," says Comes. "Because of that approach, we really didn't get a lot of pushback."

One of the significant challenges in building brands across a large health system is that often, different parts of the organization have different cultures, either because they were acquired along the way or because of the type of service they provide. For example, outpatient clinics or same-day surgery centers often have a different approach to service than inpatient units at hospitals. Part of Ascension Health, the nation's largest nonprofit Catholic health system, the Borgess Health system includes a 424-bed medical center, with a medical staff of more than 600 physicians, a 25-bed critical care access hospital, a 43-bed long-term acute care hospital, a 121-bed nursing home, and numerous clinics, outpatient facilities, a free-standing health and fitness center, and more. Because Borgess Health follows a unified brand naming hierarchy (with all entities using "Borgess" in the name), it's important to deliver a consistent brand experience across the system.

The head of the system's ambulatory care division left in the middle of the brand strategy process, leaving that group without a voice at the table during a critical juncture in the process. Although it couldn't be helped at the time, Comes wishes they could have had someone from that area committed until the end. Without that involvement, it's taken more work to show this group how the brand promise extends to their realm, beyond the inpatient settings of the medical center or critical care access hospital. The challenge is also difficult, he says, because they are physically separated from the main facilities, making it harder to reinforce the brand values on a day-to-day basis.

As with the vast majority of healthcare provider organizations, the lack of understanding of brand was widespread at Borgess. When rolling out the brand strategy in the organization, says Comes, it was a constant challenge to communicate the value of the work. One key to overcoming this challenge was showing employees how they could support the brand promise in what they do as part of their everyday jobs. Comes and his team use numerous stories and case histories to demonstrate what living the brand can mean. Brand values also are communicated through an orientation video for new employees, the organization's marketing communications vehicles, and "Borgess Brand Brief," a periodic internal publication. The Brief reinforces brand embodiment through patient stories, employee recognition, and statistics, and features perspectives on branding from outside the healthcare industry.

The challenge of the branding learning curve also presented itself during the process to develop the brand strategy, says Comes.

"Most marketers breathe branding, but others in healthcare live in a totally different world," he says. "You can't assume they know this stuff and just dive in. They are very process-oriented, and need to move step by step. It may sound funny, but the more 'process' you can build into the process, the better."

For example, he says, it was helpful to prepare for every meeting and lay out specifically what would be covered, then to follow up immediately with a recap and next steps. Because most of the participants are overwhelmed with their everyday duties, Comes notes, it was critical to set up the process right so that when they were on hand to participate, they were fully engaged. Once they left those meetings, he says, most would quickly move away from the brand process and become absorbed in their own worlds.

As is common in processes involving the consideration of such esoteric concepts as "brand," the group would often get caught up on what might seem like the smallest of details. For example, the group was considering the brand value of *restore*, and some participants had different opinions on what the word meant, whereas others feared that *restore* amounted to a guarantee of improved health, which they obviously couldn't give. Other discussions took place over words such as *optimal* and *innovation*, which had to be redefined for many as something related to more than just technology.

"Like every other healthcare provider in the world, I'd guess, we wanted to include 'caring,' " laughs Comes. "That's fine, as long as we remember that caring is just the price of admission for a healthcare brand. It's a given, it's not enough."

Comes advises patience to those embarking on a brand strategy development process. Given the deep concepts of branding, the steep learning curve for many, and the importance of the work, he says, it can be a difficult journey. This is one reason that having a strong outside partner is so important, he suggests.

"If you're looking for a formula, you will get frustrated. The process is intuitive, and it's very hard for people to know what to expect until they can see it and feel it at the other end," he says. "You just have to trust, and hold hands all the way through."

But as with others who have made it out on the other side, it can be exciting to see how the brand is brought to life.

"I've never really been a part of something like this before," he says, "where we're actually doing what we set out to do."

Case study: Mayo Clinic

For proof that an organization has a brand whether it's pursuing branding or not, look no further than the Mayo Clinic. The organization has been arguably the best-known and highest-valued healthcare system for more than a century. More than 521,000 unique patients visited a Mayo Clinic facility in 2006, and the organization took in more than $5.2 billion in patient revenues that year. It routinely ranks at the top of reputational surveys, such as the annual "Best Hospitals" ranking by *U.S. News & World Report*, and in a survey of U.S. consumers was cited (unaided) by nearly 19% of respondents as the first choice for care in the nation, nearly three times the next healthcare provider listed. Yet the organization has never run mass brand advertising. Only recently has it used a limited amount of specific advertising. More telling is the fact that it didn't begin to apply brand management explicitly as a strategy until the mid-1990s.

A cultural foundation

Of course, folks at the Mayo Clinic will say that the organization has been building its brand from the beginning, when brothers William J. Mayo and Charles H. Mayo started treating patients in Rochester, MN, in 1863. And they would be right, because as discussed earlier, brands are built primarily from the experience delivered by a product, service, or organization. So, when branding first entered the corporate vernacular in the 1990s at the Mayo Clinic, leaders were blessed with an already extraordinarily strong brand. Just as the brand was first built through the care delivered by the two Mayo brothers, the organization still considers its people the number-one way to uphold and build its powerful brand.

"We honestly believe that what makes Mayo Clinic great, what sets us apart, is our people," says Amy Davis, chair of the Mayo Clinic's Brand Team. "They are the ones creating our brand."

In a service organization, the employees themselves are often at the center of the brand experience. The question becomes, how does an organization align its employees with the desired brand promise? As I've noted, it starts with understanding at a basic level what the desired brand promise is, or how the organization wants to be valued by those it serves. At the center of it all for the Mayo Clinic is the brand promise "the needs of the patients come first." The promise is further supported by a set of principles called the Model of Care. The Model of Care is broken down into 14 core values, such as "Respect for the patient, family, and the patient's local physician."

"Sometimes it's hard for those who don't work here to understand, but rarely do you go through a day without hearing these ideas in a meeting or in a conversation," says Davis. "When we're making decisions, we'll constantly ask: 'What's best for the patient?', because if you don't walk the walk and actually use these values every day in making decisions, it won't matter. Brand values can't just be words on a wall."

Because the Mayo Clinic brand is rooted in its culture, the organization often uncovers new ways to build on its brand that bubble up from the people, as opposed to always having to drive change down from the top.

"I'm amazed all the time by things I see, and think 'Wow—was that even intentional?' " says Thomas "Tripp" Welch, who serves as section head for Workforce Research in the Mayo Clinic's Department of Human Resources. "But whether it was intended strategically or not is beside the point, because with the right culture in place, great things can come from anywhere."

Reinforcing the message

Employees are exposed to the Model of Care and core brand values from day one, starting with a two-day orientation program. New hires hear stories, learn the history of the Mayo Clinic, and review the mission and vision statements, as well as hear inspiring stories about the Model of Care. Twelve weeks following the orientation, new hires participate in a second follow-up session, where culture and legacy are further reinforced and where they have an opportunity to ask questions to a panel of Mayo leaders.

According to Welch, reinforcing the desired brand experience is a never-ending effort. Every employee's job description starts with concepts such as "teamwork," "integrity," and "compassion," and performance reviews focus on these and other core values. The organization offers many continuing education and professional development opportunities, including a series on "culture and heritage." The organization has an annual week-long Heritage Celebration, and even has Heritage Hall, a museum dedicated to the people and stories that have made the Mayo Clinic so unique over the years.

The organization is also careful about how its brand is leveraged. Although a detailed set of brand management guidelines exists, the choices aren't always easy. For example, many Mayo Clinic physicians and scientists are inventors, and they, along with the Mayo Clinic, want to take those discoveries to market to positively affect people around the world. At the same time, healthcare consumers can be distrustful of the medical technology and pharmaceutical companies who help to bring these discoveries to market and who are perceived to financially influence healthcare decisions. For the Mayo Clinic, this is a brand management balancing act. Putting the Mayo Clinic name on discoveries that positively affect people around the world represents the organization's innovation and commitment to health and humanity. But associating the Mayo Clinic with such a commercial industry is also a risk. The organization puts legal provisions for use of its name in every legal contract to carefully protect how its name and brand are used in the market to protect the strong integrity values inherent in its brand.

Making branding accessible internally

Davis, Welch, and others at the Mayo Clinic charged with driving brand embodiment are careful in how they broach the idea of branding internally. For starters, they rarely if ever use the term *internal brand* to describe this work.

"The values that appear in the Model of Care, or in the job descriptions, for example, are absolutely brand values," says Welch. "We refer to them as brand values in our brand management conversations, but we don't use that terminology out in the organization. For people to really get this, we need to use language they can relate to."

Instead, says Welch, they use terms such as *culture* and *experience* to describe brand embodiment internally. He says there was no legitimate need to use the word *brand* to encourage these efforts; instead, it was natural and more effective to continue to use words such as *experience*, which had been in use for decades and which employees intuitively understood.

"It doesn't matter who you are—physician, administrator, nurse—the core value is that patients come first," says Davis. "There's no reason to mess with that clarity just to use branding terminology."

Choosing the right words to demonstrate the Mayo Clinic brand is important in other ways as well. For example, Davis says that when the Model of Care was first developed, a 20-page brochure was created to help employees understand the purpose of the values. However, Davis says that the brochure didn't inspire employees. And the Mayo Clinic believes strongly in inspiring employees about where they work.

"The content in the Model of Care is meaningful, but it's hard to make it inspiring through a lengthy definition," she says. "We wanted to avoid having it sound like the teacher's voice in the Charlie Brown cartoons—wah wah wah wah. So, we decided to use short stories to really hit it home."

Davis says the group learned from the initial text-heavy brochure, and now the Model of Care is brought to life through storytelling. For example, a storybook was produced that includes a 300-word real-life story for each value in the Model of Care, which is provided to all new hires as part of orientation (and is also often given to potential recruits). A video companion, full of inspiring stories from patient and employee perspectives, was also created. Stories have become the cornerstone of the organization's brand-building efforts.

"In healthcare, data rules, and storytelling isn't always natural for folks," says Davis. "But we've been very conscious of moving away from 'committee-speak' and using stories to demonstrate how individuals can live the Mayo Clinic brand."

Measuring brand efforts

Brand leaders also spend a lot of effort measuring the organization's delivery on its brand values, from both an external and an internal perspective. For example, Welch says employee surveys are conducted throughout the organization to see how changes are impacting employees' ability to deliver on the brand promise. He says one important aspect of these surveys is to create a feedback loop, so those who are surveyed see the results and are empowered to address any issues that are raised.

From an external perspective, brand measurement falls to the Brand Team, a committee of 16 cross-functional leaders responsible for brand management at the Mayo Clinic. Although they conduct many measurements, perhaps the most meaningful is how the group tracks the impact of the Mayo Clinic brand on word of mouth. Many research studies have shown that when it comes to making healthcare decisions, consumers rely most on the recommendations of friends and family members, more than on even physician recommendations (and certainly more than on the basis of brand advertising!). At the Mayo

Clinic, they carefully track word of mouth related to their brand through extensive patient interviews. For example, their research shows:

- Ninety-five percent of patients said "good things" about the Mayo Clinic after visits

- Those patients told an average of 46 people "good things" about the Mayo Clinic

- Ninety percent of patients recommend the Mayo Clinic

- Patients recommended an average of 20 other people to the Mayo Clinic

- Of those receiving a recommendation, seven actually came to the Mayo Clinic

Using this information, brand leaders can discern that with an average of 500,000 unique patients per year, 95% speak positively to an average of 46 people, which multiplies to a reach of 21,850,000. All from word of mouth, all from the embodiment of a meaningful brand experience.

Reference

Berry, Leonard L., and Kent Seltman. "Building a Strong Services Brand: Lessons from Mayo Clinic"; *www.sciencedirect.com*, p. 1.